THE MECHANISM
AND MANAGEMENT
OF HEADACHE

The Mechanism and Management of HEADACHE

Second Edition

James W. Lance

M.D., F.R.C.P., F.R.A.C.P.

Chairman, Division of Neurology,
The Prince Henry and Prince of Wales Hospitals, Sydney;
Associate Professor of Medicine,
The University of New South Wales, Sydney, Australia

London : Butterworths

ENGLAND: BUTTERWORTH & CO. (PUBLISHERS) LTD.
                LONDON: 88 Kingsway, WC2 6AB

AUSTRALIA: BUTTERWORTHS PTY. LTD.
                SYDNEY: 586 Pacific Highway, NSW 2067
                MELBOURNE: 343 Little Collins Street, 3000
                BRISBANE: 240 Queen Street, 4000

CANADA: BUTTERWORTH & CO. (CANADA) LTD.
                TORONTO: 14 Curity Avenue, 374

NEW ZEALAND: BUTTERWORTHS OF NEW ZEALAND LTD.
                WELLINGTON: 26–28 Waring Taylor Street, 1

SOUTH AFRICA: BUTTERWORTH & CO. (SOUTH AFRICA) (PTY.) LTD.
                DURBAN: 152–154 Gale Street

15.3 73

Suggested U.D.C. Number: 616.831—009.7
Suggested Additional Numbers: 616.857

ISBN 0 407 26456 6

Printed in Great Britain by
Bell & Bain Ltd.
Glasgow

To my wife
and our five young headaches, whose
mechanism and management are beyond me

Contents

Preface to the Second Edition

In the three years since the appearance of the first edition sufficient research work has been done on vascular headache to warrant considerable revision of the text. The greatest changes have taken place in the understanding of migraine, particularly the nature of hormonal influences on premenstrual migraine and the mechanism of action of new pharmaceutical agents for the control of migraine. Cluster headache (migrainous neuralgia) has now been culled from the migrainous fold and granted the dignity of a chapter to itself. Minor alterations have been made throughout the book to bring each section into line with current thought. Seventy references have been added, but 57 have been deleted to preserve the quality of ease of reading. References have been removed not because they are necessarily outdated but because, for the most part, they were essential for the documentation of facts which are now generally accepted. The author hopes that the new text has gained in authority, while remaining comfortable to hold lightly in one hand.

Sydney, N.S.W.   JAMES W. LANCE

Preface to the First Edition

About once a month, until the age of 70 years, George Bernard Shaw suffered a devastating headache which lasted for a day. One afternoon, after recovering from an attack, he was introduced to Nansen and asked the famous Arctic explorer whether he had ever discovered a headache cure.

'No,' said Nansen with a look of amazement.

'Have you ever tried to find a cure for headaches?'

'No.'

'Well, that is a most astonishing thing!' exclaimed Shaw. 'You have spent your life in trying to discover the North Pole, which nobody on earth cares tuppence about, and you have never attempted to discover a cure for the headache, which every living person is crying aloud for.'[118]

It is easy for a person who has never been troubled with headaches to lose patience with those who are plagued by them. The reaction of the virtuous observer may pass through a phase of sympathetic concern to one of frustrated tolerance and, finally, to a mood of irritation and resentment in which the recurrence of headaches is attributed to a defective personality or escape from unpleasant life situations. The sound sleeper is traditionally intolerant of the insomniac and the speedy of bowel is just a little contemptuous of the constipated. In short, we tend to consider ourselves as the norm and to look quizzically at those whose physiological or psychological processes are at variance with our own. Such an attitude often persists in spite of years of advanced education and scientific training. To make it clear that I am not numbering myself among the righteous, I must state that I am not subject to headache and that my spirits often sink when confronted with a succession of patients whose contorted expressions testify to a lifetime of headache misery. This is about the only circumstance which I find likely to provoke headache in myself—I suppose on the principle that, if you can't beat them, join them!

It would be foolish to deny that the workings of the mind are of great importance in the production of headache, but they are only part of the story.

My interest in migraine was first aroused when working at the Northcott Neurological Centre in Sydney. Each patient with migraine gave a history that was a little different from the others but all were variations on a clearly recognizable theme. It seemed that all the clues were there to point the way to the understanding of the mechanism of migraine. These thoughts led to studies of the clinical features and natural history of migraine and, later, to laboratory work which now suggests that migraine is an hereditary recurrent metabolic disturbance. If this be the case, a patient cannot be held responsible for having migraine attacks any more than a woman for having menstrual periods. The treatment of migraine has improved with better understanding of the syndrome but knowledge of the migraine mechanism and its treatment still leave much to be desired.

Mysteries remain in the problem of tension headache although the place of psychological factors is much more obvious in this group than in migraine and an association with chronic over-contraction of muscle is almost universal. However, many tense, frowning people do not get headaches and the explanation for those that do must go beyond a catalogue of undesirable personality traits and bad luck in cards or love. Migraine and tension headache are given most space in this small book because they are common complaints, not always easy to diagnose and treat, and which worry patients and their medical attendants. Other common forms of headache such as those arising from eyestrain or sinusitis are not emphasized as much, because their mechanism and management are more straightforward. Serious acute headaches which betoken some hazardous intracranial condition are described sufficiently to assist in diagnosis, but not dealt with at length since their management usually becomes the prerogative of the specialist neurological unit.

This book is designed to be relatively easy armchair reading for the general practitioner, senior medical student or others who may be interested in the mechanism of headache or be concerned with the

xii

practical management of headache problems. The neurologist may find something of interest in the chapters on tension headache and migraine. References are listed for those who wish to read in greater depth.

The present concept of headache mechanisms depends to a great extent on the work of the late Harold G. Wolff and his colleagues, which is described in Wolff's monograph *Headache and other Head Pain*. The reader is referred to this work for aspects of headache which are passed over lightly here. The subject may not have all the excitement of a detective story but the talents of the great detectives of fiction would not be lost in trying to unravel some of the complexities of headache.

J. W. L.

Acknowledgements

The biochemical studies in migraine which are described in this book were undertaken by Donald A. Curran, M.D., Michael Anthony, M.D. and Brian Somerville, M.D., during the tenure of a research fellowship in neurology provided by Sandoz (Australia) Ltd., in the author's department. The research programme owes much to the advice and help of Herta Hinterberger, Ph.D., Senior Research Officer, and Robert Bartholomew, Ph.D., director of the Division of Clinical Chemistry, The Prince Henry Hospital, Sydney, and is being continued by Dr. Anthony. I am grateful to my neurosurgical colleagues Dr. A. Gonski, Dr. J. L. Dowling and Dr. B. R. Selecki for years of friendly collaboration in managing headache and other problems.

I wish to thank my secretary, Mrs. R. M. Kendall, for her willing and efficient assistance, which always makes my tasks a lot lighter. My thanks are also due to Miss B. Pate, Librarian, for obtaining all references.

The anatomical diagrams were made by Mr. J. Elliott Watson of the School of Anatomy, University of New South Wales, and the line drawings by Mrs G. Lindley. All photographs and figures were prepared by the Department of Medical Illustration, University of New South Wales.

I am grateful to the editors of the following publications for permission to reproduce figures from some of my earlier papers: *Medical Journal of Australia; Journal of Neurology, Neurosurgery and Psychiatry; Archives of Neurology; Research and Clinical Studies in Headache* (Karger of Basel and New York); *Headache* and the *Journal of Neurological Sciences.* Figures are reproduced from

ACKNOWLEDGEMENTS

Dr. Somerville's papers on hormonal changes in migraine by courtesy of the editors of *Neurology*.

The editors and publishers of *The Cellular and Molecular Basis of Neurologic Disease* have given me permission to use in this book material provided by myself and Dr. Michael Anthony for Chapter 101 of their publication.

1—Causes of Headache

A CONSIDERATION OF PAIN PATHWAYS AND GENERAL MECHANISMS OF HEADACHE

The question 'why does the head ache?' is not as naïve as it appears at first. The brain, the ependymal lining of the ventricles and choroid plexuses within the brain and much of the dura and pia-arachnoid which cover the convexity of the brain are insensitive to pain. The floor of the anterior and posterior fossa gives rise to pain on stimulation but the middle cranial fossa is sensitive only in the vicinity of the middle meningeal artery. Direct pressure on cranial nerves which carry pain fibres will of course give rise to pain, but this is an uncommon event. The most important structures which register intra cranial pain are the vessels, particularly the proximal part of the cerebral and dural arteries, and the large veins and venous sinuses.[153] A fever or 'hangover' gives rise to a throbbing headache because the cerebral arteries are dilated. An expanding lesion in one hemisphere (for example haematoma, abscess or tumour) produces headache by displacing vessels, often pushing the anterior cerebral arteries across the midline. Rapid enlargement of the ventricles, caused by internal hydrocephalus from obstruction of the cerebrospinal fluid (CSF) pathways, thrusts vessels outwards symmetrically. Oedema of the cerebral hemispheres displaces centrally placed vessels inwards as well, since the ventricles become smaller because of pressure from the swollen brain. When the pressure of CSF, which helps maintain the brain in its normal position, is lowered by lumbar puncture, the brain may pull on its supporting structures and cause headache by traction on the intracranial vessels. Because of their vascular origin, all forms of intracranial headache tend to throb with the pulse, more especially on exertion, and are made worse by any sudden jolt or jar, or with coughing, sneezing or straining.

1

Pain from the Dura

Pain from the upper surface of the tentorium and the anterior and middle cranial fossae is transmitted by the trigeminal nerve. A recurrent branch of the trigeminal nerve arises from the first (ophthalmic) division near its origin and supplies the superior surface of the tentorium and the falx, so that pain from vessels in these areas of dura is readily referred to the eye and forehead of the same side. Afferent fibres from the middle meningeal artery are of trigeminal origin, mainly from the second and third divisions.[134] The tentorium is the watershed for dural innervation since its inferior surface and the whole of the posterior fossa is supplied chiefly by the upper three cervical nerve roots and so refers pain to the back of the head and upper part of the neck. The ninth and tenth cranial nerves supply part of the posterior fossa and thus pain may sometimes be referred to the ear or throat. The result of the innervation of the dura and its vessels, in brief, is that pain from supratentorial structures is referred to the anterior two-thirds of the head by the trigeminal nerve and pain from infratentorial structures is referred to the back of the head and neck by the upper cervical nerve roots (*Figures 1.1 and 1.2*).

Pain from Cerebral Arteries

Apart from the vessels of the dura, the larger proximal parts of the intracerebral arteries are sensitive to stimulation and refer pain to the eye, forehead or temple of the same side.[68] During carotid angiography under local anaesthesia, the injection of contrast medium into the internal carotid artery is signalled by pain felt deeply behind the eye. The pain of intracranial vascular headache induced by histamine depends upon the integrity of the trigeminal nerve.[150] Blood pressure responses elicited in the monkey by stimulating the vicinity of cortical arteries are abolished by section of the trigeminal nerve.[201] It therefore seems logical that pain from the intracranial arteries is mediated in some way by the trigeminal nerve but the pathway concerned remains an anatomical puzzle.

The nerve plexus which surrounds the internal and external carotid systems in man is almost entirely of sympathetic origin from the eighth cervical and the first, second and third thoracic segments of the spinal cord via the superior cervical ganglion. There is a small parasympathetic contribution from the facial nerve through the greater superficial petrosal nerve.[42] Both internal and external carotid nerve plexuses contain some myelinated fibres of larger calibre than

2

those of sympathetic origin, which are thought to be afferent fibres of the vagus nerve and upper thoracic spinal nerves.[111,112] In the region of the carotid sinus, the internal carotid plexus receives twigs from the third, fourth and sixth cranial nerves, but there is no evidence of any constant communication with the fifth (trigeminal)

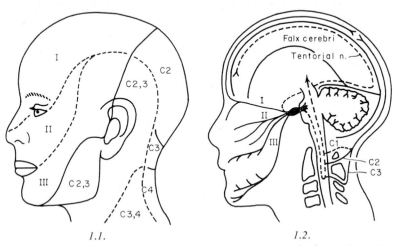

1.1.   *1.2.*

Figure 1.1. Cutaneous distribution of the trigeminal nerve to the face and anterior two-thirds of the scalp, showing the watershed with the cervical nerves above the ear line (after Cunningham)

Figure 1.2. Schematic representation of the three divisions of the trigeminal nerve, the Gasserian ganglion and the upper cervical nerve roots. Attention is drawn to three interrupted lines. One line indicates the path taken by the spinal tract and nucleus of the trigeminal nerve as it descends into the upper cervical segments of the cord. Afferent fibres from the first, second and third cervical nerve roots and the trigeminal pathway converge upon some cells in the posterior horns of the spinal cord, thus permitting referral of pain from neck to head and vice versa. The crossed second order neurones pass upwards to the thalamus. Another interrupted line indicates the course of the tentorial nerve. The first cervical nerve root is represented by an interrupted line because it is inconstant

nerve to account for the distribution of pain from the internal carotid artery and its branches to the anterior part of the head.[67] There is clinical evidence that some pain fibres from these vessels may take a long route home by descending in the peri-vascular plexus and then accompanying sympathetic nerve fibres to the upper thoracic and lower cervical spinal cord. Fay[68] described headache persisting in spite of division of the trigeminal, glossopharyngeal and vagal nerves as well as the upper three cervical nerve roots. The headache which survived such extensive surgical measures finally disappeared when spinal anaesthesia was induced and extended upwards until it

3

involved the eighth cervical segment with the onset of numbness on the ulnar aspects of the hands. This supports the anatomical evidence of afferent fibres descending in the carotid plexus to enter the spinal cord, but the part which these play in the appreciation of vascular headache has not been established.

The vertebral arterial plexus is less constant than that of the carotid system. Fang[67] demonstrated that innervation was solely unilateral in over two-thirds of human subjects. Small contributions to the vertebrobasilar plexus are made from the third, fifth, seventh, ninth, eleventh and twelfth cranial nerves.

Pain from Extracranial Arteries

The scalp arteries comprise the supra-orbital, frontal, superficial temporal, postauricular and occipital arteries, all of which receive filaments from adjacent cutaneous nerves. Ray and Wolff[153] showed that these arteries were sensitive to stimulation and stretching and were able to produce a throbbing headache by rhythmically distending and collapsing the superficial temporal artery. If several portions of the artery were distended together, the subject became nauseated. When the nerves around the scalp arteries were blocked with a local anaesthetic agent, the whole vessel did not become numb, indicating that there were multiple sources of nerve supply to the artery throughout its length. Pain is experienced in the immediate neighbourhood of an artery which is inflamed or distended. Pain from the supra-orbital, frontal and superficial temporal arteries is mediated by the trigeminal nerve, and from the postauricular and occipital arteries by the upper cervical nerve roots.

Pain from the Skull, Sinuses, Eyes, Teeth and Neck

The cranial bones are insensitive, but stretch of the periosteum evokes pain locally. Pain from the eye, nasal sinuses and teeth is felt locally at first, then may be referred to the appropriate division of the trigeminal nerve, with some overflow to adjacent divisions if the pain is severe. Diffuse headache from contraction of head and neck muscles may follow later if local pain is sustained. The whole pattern then assumes the character of tension headache and muscular overaction can be demonstrated by electromyography.[214]

Degenerative changes in the upper cervical spine may cause compression of the first, second and third cervical nerve roots with referral of pain to the back of the head. Pain from a cervical disc lesion may rarely be referred to one eye and one half of the head,

4

probably because some afferent fibres from the first and second cervical nerve roots converge upon cells in the posterior horn of the spinal cord, which can also be excited by trigeminal afferent fibres,[101] thus conveying to the patient the impression of head pain through this shared pathway. Stimulation of the first, but not the second, cervical posterior root consistently gives rise to frontal and orbital pain in man.[102] Wolff mentions that the second and third nerve roots may refer pain to the vertex. There is no known way for lesions of the lower cervical spine to cause pain in the head other than by producing overaction of the head and neck muscles, presumably in a subconscious or reflex attempt to prevent neck movement.

Muscle-contraction or 'tension' headache can be relieved by the infiltration of local anaesthetic into the affected muscle and is mediated by the trigeminal nerve or the upper cervical nerve roots.

Central Pathways for Head Pain

Pain fibres from all three divisions of the trigeminal nerve descend in a laminated arrangement as the spinal tract of the fifth nerve down to the second cervical segment of the spinal cord. They are joined in their path by pain fibres from the facial, glossopharyngeal and vagus nerves which also plunge down into the spinal cord. Recent work has shown that the intraspinal portion of the descending trigeminal tract and nucleus in the upper two segments of the cervical cord is the main relay centre for pain from the head.[103] Sensory fibres from the upper three cervical dorsal roots ramify throughout this centre and make some synaptic contact with trigeminal neurones in the spinal nucleus, which permits referral of pain from the upper neck to the head and vice versa (see Figure 1.2). After synapsing, the second order neurones cross the midline and ascend through the brainstem as the quinto-thalamic tract to the posteroventromedial nucleus of the thalamus. That there is considerable interaction between trigeminal and cervical volleys was shown by Denny-Brown and Yanagisawa[58] in the monkey. They were able to show both inhibitory and excitatory effects from the cervical segments on trigeminal function, the inhibitory effects being reversed by the use of strychnine.

SUMMARY

The scalp vessels, cranial periosteum and dura are innervated chiefly by the trigeminal nerve over the anterior two-thirds of the head, and by the upper three cervical nerve roots over the posterior third.

5

Displacement or dilatation of intracranial vessels and distension of extracranial arteries are common causes of headache. It is not certain which pain pathways serve the sensitive basal portion of the intra-cranial arteries, although the areas to which pain is referred are in the trigeminal distribution. There is evidence that some pain fibres descend with the periarterial nerve plexuses in the neck to reach the lower cervical and upper thoracic spinal cord, but the role of these fibres in headache is uncertain.

Overlap between the projection of afferent fibres in the upper cervical nerve roots and those of the trigeminal nerve offer an explanation for the referral of pain to the head in disorders of the upper cervical spine.

2—Varieties of Headache and their Classification

The consideration of pain pathways and mechanisms involved in the perception of headache leads naturally to thoughts on the classification of headache. Headache may be divided into groups on the grounds of site, acuteness of onset, association with neurological signs and many other clinical criteria. Such categories help in differential diagnosis and will be used for this purpose later on. The most useful classification of the many varieties of headache to precede individual clinical descriptions is one which is based as far as possible on knowledge of pain mechanisms. The classification presented here is modified from the recommendations of the Ad Hoc Committee on Classification of Headache[74] by consolidation and rearrangement of some categories in an attempt to make it more easily understood by those who are not completely familiar with the subject and to make it easier to remember the main headings for those who wish to do so.

Intracranial Sources of Headache

(1) Meningeal irritation, as in subarachnoid haemorrhage, meningitis, encephalitis or post-pneumoencephalographic reaction.

(2) Traction on, or displacement of, intracranial vessels. This may be due to:

  (a) space-occupying lesions, such as tumour, haematoma or abscess;

  (b) increased intracranial pressure, for example blockage of CSF pathways (hydrocephalus), superior sagittal or lateral sinus thrombosis (otitic hydrocephalus), raised venous pressure (emphysema, mediastinal obstruction), cerebral oedema from other causes (malignant hypertension, 'benign intracranial hypertension', hypocalcaemia, adrenal corticosteroids, Addison's disease); or

(c)   reduced intracranial pressure, as in post lumbar puncture headache.

(3)   Simple intracranial vasodilatation, the cause of which may be

(a)   toxic, for example systemic infections, 'hangover', carbon monoxide poisoning, caffeine withdrawal, foreign protein reactions;

(b)   metabolic, for example hypoxia, hypoglycaemia, hypercapnia;

(c)   vasodilator drugs, such as histamine or nitrites;

(d)   post-concussional;

(e)   post-convulsive;

(f)   acute cerebral vascular insufficiency;

(g)   acute pressor reactions, such as acute nephritis, phaeochromocytoma, tyramine ingestion by a patient taking monoamine oxidase inhibitors; or

(h)   early morning headache of hypertension.

(4)   Exertional and cough headache of benign aetiology.

Extracranial Vascular Headache

(1)   Vascular headache of migraine type, which may be common migraine, classic migraine, basilar artery migraine, hemiplegic migraine, ophthalmoplegic migraine, facial migraine ('lower half headache').

(2)   Cluster headache, lower half headache, migrainous neuralgia.

(3)   Inflammation of extracranial vessels, for example giant cell arteritis.

Muscle-contraction Headache

(1)   Secondary to other factors, as in eyestrain, imbalance of bite, cervical spondylosis.

(2)   Primary muscle overaction (tension headache).

(3)   Combination with extracranial vascular headache (tension vascular headache).

Cranial Nerve Disorders

(1) Compression or inflammation of cranial nerves.
(2) Trigeminal and glossopharyngeal neuralgia.
(3) Excessive stimulation (ice-cream headache).

Local Cranial Disorders

(1) Expanding lesion within cranial bone stretching periosteum.
(2) Inflammation of cranium or scalp.

Referred Pain

(1) Eyes, as in increased intra-ocular pressure, inflammation.
(2) Ears, nose and throat, as in sinusitis, nasopharyngeal carcinoma.
(3) Teeth, for example root abscess.
(4) Neck, for example cervical spondylosis.

Psychogenic Headache

Depressive, delusional, conversion or hypochondriacal states.

Atypical Facial Pain

Commonly associated with a depressive state, but mechanism not understood.

Post-Traumatic Headaches

These comprise an important aetiological category but their mechanism embraces vascular, neural and psychological factors which could lead to their classification under a number of the above headings.

3—Recording the History

The diagnostic battle is often lost or won in the first skirmish. If a patient complaining of headache or facial pain is first seen in a busy office or general clinic, with a background noise of coughing and shuffling feet from the waiting room, it is probably better to make an appointment for another time when the problem can be discussed in detail. If sufficient time is given to the initial interview, the majority of patients can be assessed adequately without recourse to special investigations. A careful systematic history will enable one to make a firm diagnosis of some disorders such as cluster headache and tic douloureux and to make a provisional diagnosis in most patients with tension headache, migraine, sinusitis, ocular disturbance or cervical spondylosis. The evolution of the headache may raise suspicions of more serious conditions such as subdural haematoma, cerebral tumour or temporal arteritis. The history is much more important than physical examination, which is often completely normal in patients with headache.

The most convenient form for the history is the same as that used to gather information about pain elsewhere in the body. When the essential points are always written down in the same order under the same headings, a pattern of headache emerges in the shortest possible time which is often sufficient to make the diagnosis. The writing of a long narrative in the rambling or disconnected sequence dictated by a loquacious patient is an interesting literary exercise for those with time on their hands. It has the disadvantage that the diagnostic pattern of the story may be obscured and that if the patient should be subject to more than one kind of headache, the strands of each may become hopelessly interwoven in the verbal loom.

The following excerpt from the casebook of a well-known physician makes some important points but is not complete enough to permit of diagnosis with certainty:

> Most of the time he seemed to see something shining before him like a light, usually in part of the right eye; at the end of a moment, a violent pain supervened in the right temple, then in all the head and neck, where the head is attached to the spine . . . vomiting, when it became possible, was able to divert the pain and render it more moderate.

A more elaborate description of a headache syndrome, written in discursive style, still omits information which we would like to have:

> In certain cases, the parts on the right side, or those on the left solely, so far that a separate temple, or ear, or one eyebrow, or one eye, or the nose which divides the face into two equal parts; and the pain does not pass this limit, but remains in the half of the head. This is called Heterocrania, an illness by no means mild, even though it intermits and although it appears to be slight. For if at any time it set in acutely, it occasions unseemly and dreadful symptoms; spasm and distortion of the countenance takes place; the eyes either fixed intently like horns, or they are rolled inwardly to this side or to that; vertigo, deep-seated pain of the eyes as far as the meninges; irrestrainable sweat; sudden pain of the tendons, as of one striking with a club; nausea; vomiting of bilious matters; collapse of the patient . . . there is much torpor, heaviness of the head, anxiety, and ennui. For they flee the light; the darkness soothes their disease: nor can they bear readily to look upon or hear anything agreeable; their sense of smell is vitiated, neither does anything agreeable to smell delight them; and they have also an aversion to fetid things: The patients, moreover, are weary of life, and wish to die.

The first description was written by Hippocrates[44] about 400 B.C. and the second by Aretaeus of Cappadocia[2] about A.D. 150. The vividness of imagery leaves little doubt that both were depicting migraine, although other disorders may have crept in to Aretaeus' account. Since the average medical man is not writing his case histories for posterity, greater economy of style may be granted to him and a systematic record will give a clearer, if less elegant, picture of the patient's illness. It is often of assistance to quote directly any phrase of the patient's which appears well-chosen and likely to throw light on the illness.

There would still be notable gaps in the record of these headaches of antiquity if the above quotations were combined and transcribed in summary, as follows;

Length of illness: unstated
Frequency of headache: unstated

Duration of headache:	unstated
Site of headache:	half head, right or left, maximal in temple, eye or frontal region, radiating to ear, nostril and neck.
Quality of headache:	'violent' (constant or pulsating?)
Time of onset:	unstated
Mode of onset:	light shining in part of right eye (in right half of visual field?) lasting a moment
Associated features:	nausea, vomiting, photophobia, disturbed sense of smell, sweating, vertigo, aching limbs, anxiety, depression and drowsiness. Collapse (syncopal attack? epileptic in view of eyes rolling?)
Precipitating factors:	unstated. (We could here insert 'drinking wine ... or heat of a fire, or the sun', by borrowing from the Roman physician Cornelius Celsus, a friend of the Emperor Tiberius[44])
Relieving factors:	darkness, vomiting. Specific therapy (namely, bleeding and the use of hellebore) is mentioned elsewhere by Hippocrates[44]

This analysis gives a vivid picture of migraine (with some atypical features) but is not helpful in establishing the temporal pattern of attacks which is so important in diagnosis, and in the timing of treatment to prevent attacks. The temporal pattern also serves as a baseline on which to assess the results of therapy. If the patient is subject to bouts of headache lasting for several weeks followed by freedom from headache for months, one obviously has to be careful about interpreting a remission as the result of treatment. Lack of knowledge of the natural history of cluster headache was responsible for cures being attributed to histamine desensitization, while in fact the natural periodicity of the disorder remained unaltered by treatment. Any serious assessment of results must be controlled by the use of a placebo or an alternative treatment without the knowledge of either patient or physician of which treatment they are being given until after their response is documented. This sort of procedure is unnecessary in normal clinical practice but a healthy and critical scepticism must be maintained as any disorder fluctuates in intensity and the remission may easily be abetted by the enthusiastic adoption of a new method of treatment.

To assist diagnosis of headache and help plan treatment it is thus worthwhile to have standard headings, such as those which have just been applied impiously to Hippocrates and Aretaeus.

At the top of the history sheet, the presenting symptom may be written as:

Headaches, 6 years.

If there has been a change in pattern during the course of the illness, this is best mentioned at the onset:

Headaches 6 years, worse 2 years.

When the patient complains of two or more varieties of headache these can be nominated separately at the onset and a line drawn down the middle of the history sheet so that data for each type of headache can be set out side by side. As an example let us take the history of a hypothetical woman aged 30 years, writing down the important positive and negative features in abbreviated form.

Headaches (1) unilateral with vomiting, 6 years;
(2) dull bilateral, 2 years.

The history may be written as follows:

	Type (1)	Type (2)
Frequency:	4 every month	almost daily
Duration	1 day	most of day
Site:	frontotemporal (L or R)	bifrontal
Quality:	throbbing, then severe and constant	dull, constant pressing
Time of onset:	any time, often 4–5 a.m.	on rising
Mode of onset:	occasionally blurred vision precedes headache by 10 min.	headache only
Associated features:	nausea, vomiting, photophobia, blurred vision, bloodshot eyes no teichopsia no diplopia no paraesthesiae, paresis no dysphasia slurred speech, vertigo and ataxia at height of headache lack of concentration no faintness, loss of consciousness polyuria as headache eases	light-headed at times no other symptoms

13

Precipitating factors:	attacks more frequent with menses alcohol, fatty foods, missing a meal may trigger attacks	worse during stress at work, entertaining at home, or when children misbehave
Relieving factors	no headache for last 6 months of her two pregnancies	no change during pregnancies
	frequency unaltered by vacations	eases when on vacation
	rest and darkness ergotamine tartrate, if taken at onset, shortens attack to 2 hours no trial of interval medication	relieved for 3 hours by A.P.C. powders improved by alcohol
Pattern	Migraine	Tension headache

A clinical pattern has thus emerged of a fairly constant tension headache, punctuated by frequent attacks of migraine. Such a history is not uncommon and is a cause of considerable disability. The combination of two types of headache must be recognized at the onset to guide the taking of the remainder of the history and to point the way to effective treatment. Once the pattern of headache is established, attention is turned to the general health of the patient, with specific enquiries about symptoms of conditions which may give rise to headache.

General Health

It is important to determine at the outset whether headache is one facet of a systemic disease, or whether it may be regarded as an isolated problem.

The child who is failing to gain weight, does not look well, has altered in disposition and complains of headache, is a worrying problem. Cerebral tumour, tuberculous meningitis and blood disorders such as leukaemia may first make themselves known in this way. In some illnesses of sudden onset, there may only be a vague malaise to indicate that headache is not primarily of intracranial origin; for example, acute nephritis can present with headache, hypertension and papilloedema without urinary symptoms. On the other hand, chronic infections, collagen diseases and endocrine disorders may all have caused an unmistakable deterioration in the patient's health before the development of headache.

14

At any age impairment of general health with loss of weight raises the possibility of malignant disease. In the group aged from 55 years onwards, general malaise, loss of weight, night sweats and aching of the joints and muscles should make one think of temporal arteritis as a source of headache.

System Review

It is always helpful to ask leading questions concerning each bodily system at the conclusion of the history of the present illness. In a patient with headache, the eyes, ears, nose and throat, teeth and neck should be included in this review. The chronic obstruction of one or other nostril in vasomotor rhinitis or chronic respiratory tract infection may suggest the possibility of sinusitis. The eye may become proptosed with retro-orbital tumours or a mucocele projecting into the orbit from the frontal sinus. Dimness of vision and 'haloes' seen around lights may mark the onset of glaucoma. Complaints of impaired eyesight may draw attention to compression of the visual pathways. Papilloedema may be symptomless or the patient may notice blurring of vision on bending the head forwards. In contrast, visual loss is severe in retrobulbar neuritis and may be complete.

A space-occupying lesion or other intracranial disturbance such as progressive hydrocephalus becomes much more likely if the recent onset of headache is associated with any of the following symptoms:

Drowsiness at inappropriate times
Vomiting without apparent cause
Fits
Sudden falling attacks, in which consciousness may be retained
Progressive neurological deficit of any kind, for example, mental deterioration, impairment of senses of smell, vision or hearing. (It is remarkable how a unilateral nerve deafness may be present for years without being complained of, or even noticed, by the patient)
Double vision
Weakness or sensory impairment of the face or limbs on one or other side
Disturbed co-ordination or loss of balance, with or without vertigo
Polyuria and polydipsia
Progressive change in pituitary function. Symptoms suggesting hypopituitarism are asthenia, diminished libido, reduction of body hair, lessened shaving frequency in men, premature cessation of menstruation in women, the skin becoming soft and finely wrinkled in both sexes, and the delay of pubescence in the child. On the other hand hyperpituitarism may be responsible for excessive growth and early pubescence in the young, and deepening of the voice, enlargement of the jaw and hands in adults.

15

Past Health

A head injury at any time in the past 2 years may be of relevance. Subdural haematoma may follow a blow on the head which the patient considers trivial.

A number of episodes of 'encephalitis' or any severe headache with neck stiffness should arouse suspicions of bleeding from a cerebral angioma. A useful additional point in the history is the development of nerve-root pains in the back, buttocks and thighs some hours or days after the onset of headache, caused by blood tracking down the subarachnoid space to the cauda equina.

Any operations should be noted. The 'mole' removed 7 years ago may be the secondary melanoma of today. A past tuberculous infection may have been aroused from years of slumber.

Any debilitating illness or the use of corticosteroids may reactivate tuberculous lesions or prepare the way for cryptococcal meningitis. Recurrent renal infections or stones may underlie present hypertension. Sinusitis and recurrent ear infections are of importance, particularly in children.

Vomiting attacks and 'car-sickness' in childhood commonly precede migraine in later life. The author has always enquired after asthma, hay-fever, hives, eczema and other allergies in patients with migraine but now doubts the relevance of these questions for reasons which will become apparent in the chapter on migraine (*see Chapter 9*).

Family History

Both migraine and tension headache run in families but there is little tendency for cluster headache to do so. Information may be gained about a familial proneness to malignancy, tuberculosis, hypertension and other disorders which may relate to the problem of headache.

Personal Background

Occupation

The patient's occupation may have direct relevance to the problem of headache in the case of certain infections such as Q fever in abbattoir workers. Exposure to toxic or vasodilator substances in some chemical processes, or the tedium of a repetitive job in a noisy environment, may be responsible for headache occurring at work. The patient's interest in his occupation may have been lost for a number of reasons, perhaps the inability to see the end-result of his labour, or from the pressure of uninspired or heavy-handed management. The levelling out in middle age, when a progress assessment shows that some dreams will never be fulfilled, may cause a reaction of anxiety and depression. The waning of old skills or the difficulty in accommodating to new ideas and techniques may cast gloom over the years before retirement and when retirement finally comes it may remove an important source of motivation and take much of the zest from life.

Personal or Family Problems

The possible psychological factors which may underlie the anxiety of a child, adolescent, unmarried adult or married couple are legion. Pressure on the individual to achieve a succession of goals now starts in primary school and the goals set by parents for their children are often quite unrealistic. Feelings of inadequacy and frustration are not uncommon as a result. Statisticians would be embarrassed if every child turned out to be of above-average intelligence, personality and sporting ability.

Parental separation or divorce, or a strained marriage continuing for the sake of the children, are common causes of insecurity, tension and behaviour disturbance in childhood. It requires patient and devoted team-work between husband and wife to bring up a family successfully at the best of times.

Sexual problems may be of importance at any age. The containment within accepted social bounds of the sexual vigour of youth and the maintenance of satisfactory sexual life in marriage during the mature middle years among the tensions of work and child raising may each bring difficulties. The unmarried of any age may be troubled by the instability of their sexual and social relationships, with the spectre of loneliness at the end of the line.

All information volunteered about the patient's way of life should be considered, while bearing in mind that stress is usually insufficient in itself to cause headache. The problem lies more often in the failure of adjustment of a patient to a common situation which would not trouble most people.

Habits

The personal history also covers intake of alcohol, smoking habits and the consumption of headache powders and other drugs. The daily ingestion of up to 10 headache powders (usually containing aspirin, phenacetin and caffeine) by patients with tension headache is not uncommon and may alert the examiner to the possibility of methaemoglobinaemia or chronic renal disease from the long-continued use of analgesics. The author remembers one patient

17

C

who nibbled tablets of pentobarbitone 100 mg throughout the day 'to steady the nerves', up to a total of 12 tablets daily. She would not divulge how she obtained such liberal supplies but her habituation was a psychiatric problem in its own right.

Some proprietary relaxing agents which can be bought from a pharmacist without a prescription contain a monureide and bromide. The development of bromism with headache and confusion may be insidious.

Certain foods may precipitate a headache in susceptible people. Many migraineurs blame fatty foods, chocolates and certain fruits, particularly oranges. An interesting form of headache has recently been described in patients who have eaten a Chinese meal when monosodium glutamate has been used liberally in the preparation of the food and this has been called the Chinese restaurant syndrome.

Red wines contain tyramine and histamine which may induce migraine or other vascular headaches in a dosage lower than that usually required to produce a 'hangover'. It is said that a chronic alcoholic rarely suffers from headache and that it is advisable to think of the possibility of a subdural haematoma if he does complain of recent headaches.

Emotional State

As the personal history is taken, some insight is usually gained into whether the patient's symptoms are exaggerated by loneliness and introspection or whether they are being played down by one who has an active and interesting life. The history is a second-hand experience which is coloured by the emotional expression of the person telling the story. While the history is being recorded it may be possible to discern whether the patient reacts to problems with physical manifestations of tension by frowning, clenching the jaws or holding the head and neck rigidly. It is important to look for symptoms of depression, such as loss of interest in work, homelife or personal affairs; or staying at home and not wanting to see friends or continue with previous activities. Depressive symptoms are most important to recognize since their treatment may play a big part in restoring pleasure to life, quite apart from relieving the headache which is often a reflection of the depressive state.

4—Pattern Recognition from the History

The need for a careful and systematic history was presented in the previous chapter. The information about the headache obtained under each descriptive subheading is responsible for adding a valuable contribution to a differential diagnosis. The taking of a history is an active process. The enquiry after each aspect is like adding a chemical reagent to an unknown mixture and observing what takes place. Each step assists in the classification of headache and hence its identification.

Each subheading will be considered in turn to evaluate its significance in diagnosis or management of headache problems.

Length of Illness

The length of time for which a patient has been troubled by headache is the first guide as to whether the symptom portends some malign or progressive neurological disorder which requires further investigation. At one end of the scale, the sudden onset of severe headache, possibly followed by impairment of consciousness or focal neurological signs, suggests some serious illness such as subarachnoid haemorrhage or meningitis. At the other end of the scale, a patient who has had headaches regularly for 20, 30 or 40 years is most likely to have some form of vascular headache (migraine or one of its variants), or chronic tension (muscle-contraction) headache. The first attack of migraine which a patient experiences may be confusing unless it is preceded by characteristic symptoms, and may suggest systemic infection, encephalitis or meningitis.

19

Between the very acute and very chronic headaches lie the most difficult to interpret, those which have developed over some days, weeks or months. The subacute headache may have a relatively simple explanation such as sinusitis or some ocular cause but one must be on guard against less common but more lethal conditions such as subdural haematoma, cerebral tumour or other causes of increased intracranial pressure, or, in the age group 55–70 years, the insidious onset of temporal (giant-cell) arteritis.

Frequency and Duration of Headache

These two parameters establish the temporal pattern which is so important in the diagnosis of recurrent headache. In this group the main conditions to be considered are migraine, cluster headache, trigeminal neuralgia (tic douloureux), tension and tension-vascular headache.

Migraine may recur irregularly at intervals of months or years but commonly a pattern has become established by the time a patient seeks medical advice. The headache may be linked to the menstrual cycle or may appear one to ten times each month without any obvious cause, disappearing only during pregnancy, holidays, admission to hospital or other periods of prolonged rest. It may last from a few hours to several days, but is usually followed by a period of freedom from headache before the next attack starts.

Cluster headache, on the other hand, has an intriguing periodicity. It usually recurs in bouts lasting from 2 weeks to 3 months and then vanishes completely for 3 months to as long as 4 years. During a bout, the headache returns once, twice or three times in 24 hours, and lasts from 10 minutes to 2 hours on each occasion. The fact that the pain persists for this length of time clearly distinguishes it from trigeminal neuralgia, which recurs as transient jabs of pain, each lasting a fraction of a second, although the jabs may be repetitive. The two disorders are mentioned together because they are commonly confused in general practice. Many patients with cluster headache are referred with the provisional diagnosis of trigeminal neuralgia, probably because the pattern of cluster headache is not widely known. One point that the conditions have in common is the tendency to spontaneous remission for months or years. The distinction between the two is most important because the mechanism and treatment of each are entirely different.

Tension headache is set apart from those just considered by the absence of any paroxysmal quality or periodicity about its course. While acute forms of tension headache may appear at the end of a stressful day in a busy office or a household of screaming children,

20

the usual story of the habitué is that there is always a headache lurking in the background. Such patients have some sort of headache all day and every day. They are never really free except for an hour or two after ingestion of their favourite caffeine-containing analgesic. There is a form of headache intermediate between this undulating pattern and the paroxysms of migraine. This is termed tension-vascular headache because surges of more severe throbbing headache become superimposed every few days or weeks on an otherwise monotonous background of constant discomfort.

Site

Headache is commonly bilateral except in migraine attacks (of which about two-thirds are one-sided), cluster headache and tic douloureux (which are almost always strictly unilateral), local changes in the eye, sinuses, skull or scalp, and expanding lesions of one cerebral hemisphere. An aneurysm of the internal carotid artery may cause pain behind one eye by enlarging without rupturing. Subarachnoid haemorrhage from aneurysm or angioma may start with local pain but headache usually becomes general in distribution and spreads to the back of the neck. Space-occupying lesions may cause unilateral pain by displacement of vessels, but headache becomes bilateral if CSF pathways are obstructed. The site of headache is not reliable as a means of localizing cerebral tumour.

The headache of internal carotid thrombosis is unilateral, whereas in vertebrobasilar insufficiency pain involves the occipital area bilaterally. Scalp vessels may be involved separately in temporal arteritis so that pain is limited to the distribution of a specific artery. Less commonly, migraine headache may be limited to a particular part of the vascular tree, giving rise to frontal, temporal or occipital pain, or even involving the internal maxillary and other branches of the external carotid system to produce facial pain known as 'lower half headache'. The pain of cluster headache characteristically involves the eye and frontal region on one side and may radiate down to the nostril and cheek of the same side, overlapping the distribution of 'lower half headache'. The pain of tic douloureux is felt in one or more of the divisions of the trigeminal nerve, but starts in the first division (eye and forehead) in only 5 per cent of cases.[100]

Tension headache is usually bilateral, but may sometimes be one-sided owing to asymmetrical muscular-contraction, found particularly if there is associated imbalance of the bite. The pain of temporomandibular arthritis, resulting from an unbalanced or closed bite, may radiate in all directions from the joint in front of the ear, so that it involves much of the face and temple.

21

Quality

The most important distinction here is between pulsating or throbbing headache, indicating a vascular origin and a constant ache. Migraine commonly starts as a dull headache, soon develops a throbbing quality which then becomes a constant severe pain, possibly as the arterial wall becomes oedematous and less easily distended with each pulse. The pain of cluster headache is described as deep, boring and intense. Tic douloureux is a shock-like transient stab of intense severity. Tension headache is usually dull, constant, tight, pressing or band-like. Certain embellishments of the history may indicate hysterical characteristics ('as though my skull were going to burst into a thousand fragments'), or an obsessional personality. One patient kept a daily chart of his headaches, plotted on a scale from H1 to H10 ('you can see where my headache went up to H9: that's almost as much as a body can bear'). The severity of headache is often a quality of diagnostic significance—the pain of cluster headache, tic douloureux and some attacks of migraine may indeed approach 'H9'.

Time of Onset

Headaches resulting solely from hypertension, which are really quite uncommon, are present on waking but pass off as soon as the patient gets up and about. Migraine and tension-vascular headaches may also be present on waking or awaken the patient from sleep at 3 or 4 a.m. Cluster headache occurs by night as well as by day and frequently wakes the patient 1 or 2 hours after retiring. Tension headache does not wake the patient at night unless a vascular element becomes superimposed. The tense patient may or may not wake up free of headache but usually becomes aware of the familiar sensation as soon as the day's activities start.

The time of onset of headache is more important from the therapeutic than the diagnostic point of view. It is useless to prescribe ergotamine tartrate at the onset of a migraine attack if the patient's headache is in full bloom on waking. Medication has to be given the night before to anticipate the morning's episode. Similarly, an injection of ergotamine tartrate or an oral dose of methysergide is given on retiring to prevent nocturnal paroxysms of cluster headache.

Mode of Onset

The only form of headache with a recognizable prodrome is migraine. For 10 to 40 minutes before the headache starts there may be visual hallucinations or a complex succession of neurological

22

symptoms which adhere to much the same sequence on each occasion. Visual hallucinations may take the form of simple flashes of light or a coloured display of zig-zag scintillations (fortification spectra) moving slowly across the field leaving a scotoma behind. There may be patchy or generalized blurring of vision at the height of the disturbance or a clearly defined homonymous hemianopia.

Associated Phenomena

There are a wide variety of symptoms linked with migraine headache, including photophobia, gastrointestinal disturbance, fluid retention, and focal neurological changes, which will be discussed in detail in a later chapter.

The reddened forehead, injected conjunctiva, lacrimating eye and occasional Horner's syndrome of cluster headache are distinctive vascular phenomena. The nostril on the affected side may block or run with fluid.

The meningeal irritation of subarachnoid haemorrhage, meningitis and encephalitis causes a protective reflex muscle spasm of the extensor muscles of the neck which is manifest clinically as neck rigidity.

The sudden headache caused by a colloid cyst blocking the flow of CSF in the third ventricle may be accompanied by a 'drop attack', a sudden loss of power in the legs, caused by compression of the midline reticular formation. Consciousness is not necessarily lost with drop attacks. With any space-taking lesion, or progressive hydrocephalus, the patient may become drowsy, yawn frequently or vomit without preliminary nausea. Fits or other symptoms of focal cortical irritation may precede headache or appear as the headache intensifies. Diplopia may herald the onset of compression of the third cranial nerve, a sinister sign of an expanding intracranial mass forcing part of the temporal lobe downwards through the tentorial opening.

Rigors and sweats in any acute infectious process, nasal obstruction in sinusitis, conjunctival and circumcorneal injection in ocular conditions, are all indications of the source of headache.

Precipitating or Aggravating Factors

Any intracranial vascular headache, whether it be caused by 'hangover', hypoglycaemia or intracranial tumour, will be made worse by jarring, sudden movements of the head, coughing, sneezing or straining. 'Cough headache' is not always associated with intracranial tumour but can be a benign, if unexplained, vascular syndrome in its own right.[190] Bending the head forwards may bring on a severe paroxysmal headache in patients with colloid cyst of the third ventricle, or other forms of obstructive hydrocephalus.

Sensitivity to light is a common feature of diffuse intracranial disturbance such as meningitis or encephalitis as well as migraine. Glare, loud noises and even strong odours are liable to initiate or worsen tension headache as well as migraine.

Exercise aggravates vascular headache of any type and the occasional individual may suffer disability as a result of exercise alone. Sexual intercourse may bring on vascular or tension-vascular headaches and has been known to precipitate subarachnoid haemorrhage.

Some people are liable to a dull, vascular headache on missing a meal or several hours after a meal, and hypoglycaemia may provoke a migraine attack in susceptible patients.[24] Certain foods are said to induce migraine. There is some evidence that ingestion of tyramine-containing foods may exert a chemical influence, but doubt has been cast on whether fatty foods, chocolates, oranges and other traditional migraine precipitants act specifically or by a psychological conditioning process. Vascular reactivity appears to be altered by hormonal changes, thus accounting for the association between migraine and menstruation, and its relief in some women during pregnancy.

Alcohol usually triggers cluster headache during a bout but not at other times. It may also bring on migraine when the patient is in a susceptible phase (not in the refractory period after an attack has recently ended) and some careful observers assure the author that red wines are much more liable to do this than white.

The explosive pains of tic douloureux may be detonated by stimulation of any area served by the trigeminal nerve. Talking, chewing, swallowing, shaving or even a puff of wind blowing on to the face are trigger factors commonly mentioned. Pain arising from the teeth is usually exacerbated by hot or cold fluids in the mouth. Movement of the jaw will add a sharp quality to the pain of temporomandibular arthritis.

Changes in barometric pressure may make the pain of sinusitis worse. Anyone who has ever had a cold when travelling by air and experienced pain from the sinuses during the descent will be sufficiently impressed to carry a nasal decongestant in future. Curiously, migraine may also follow sudden changes in barometric pressure, although the reason is unknown.

The relatively uncommon headache of cervical spondylosis is understandably aggravated by neck movement, just as the muscle-contraction headache of eyestrain is brought on by reading or close

24

work. Tension headache may correlate fairly closely with periods of turbulence caused by worry, anger or excitement, but in the chronic form it may persist inexorably, no matter how calm the waters. Migraine may occur at a time of stress but it more commonly follows some hours after relaxation from stress or even the following day, as in 'weekend migraine'.

Relieving Factors

Pressure on the distended scalp arteries, or over the common carotid artery of the affected side, and the use of hot or cold compresses, are often helpful in migraine. The migrainous patient usually prefers to lie in a darkened room whereas the sufferer from cluster headache prefers to sit up or pace the floor, holding his hand over the affected eye. Rebreathing into a paper bag or the inhalation of carbon dioxide 10 per cent in air or oxygen is said to shorten the vasoconstrictive phase of migraine.

Rest is usually essential to relieve intracranial vascular headache but the early morning headache of hypertension is improved by the upright position. Headache triggered by hypoglycaemia is not necessarily relieved by the taking of food.

The pain of sinusitis is abolished when the sinuses are cleared by the relief of nasal obstruction. The avoidance of chewing on one side and excessive jaw clenching eases the pain of temporomandibular strain or arthritis until dental attention can be obtained.

Voluntary relaxation of forehead and jaw muscles will reduce the severity of tension headache and the use of alcohol or other vasodilator substances such as nicotinic acid may temporarily abolish it.

Aspirin will stop the pain of migraine in childhood but not in adult life. Aspirin continues to be useful in other mild forms of head pain. In combination with phenacetin and caffeine as A.P.C. powders it forms part of the national diet in Australia, not only for patients with tension headache but also for those who think they might get a headache if they do not take these powders.

More specific methods of relieving headache will be discussed later in the appropriate chapters.

It is to be hoped that sufficient of the factors mentioned in this chapter will emerge during the taking of a clinical history to form a clear clinical impression of the headache pattern and an opinion about the group to which the headache belongs and its probable cause. Well-directed enquiries may bring out important points which the patient has neglected to mention. If the diagnosis is not evident after taking the clinical history, at least the physician should know what to look for on physical examination and should also have formed an opinion as to whether the headache warrants further investigation.

5—*Physical Examination*

After hearing the patient's history, the physician may be alerted to look particularly carefully at certain aspects of the physical examination. In any event, the patient complaining of headache warrants a full examination. This will often be negative, but it is important to know that it is negative. The emphasis of examination will naturally be on the head and the nervous system, but there are so many ways in which headache may be produced that general examination must not be neglected.

General Appearance

The general appearance of the patient often gives some clue about the nature of the headache. The transfer of a moist handkerchief from the palm of one hand to the other, the intertwining of the fingers, the restless movements and occasional sighing respiration are indications of nervous tension as valid as the furrowed brow and periodic thrusting forward or clenching of the jaw.

The shape of the face, the size of the jaw and hands, the texture of the skin and hair, and the timbre of the voice may direct attention to the endocrine system and to the pituitary gland in particular.

If a patient is seen while suffering from cluster headache, the forehead may be flushed and conjunctival vessels dilated only on the side of the headache. A partial Horner's syndrome may be present with drooping eyelid and small pupil, and tears may be observed running from the affected eye (*Figure 5.1*). In migraine, the patient is more often pale than flushed but the conjunctivae are nonetheless

27

injected, more so on the side of the headache. Pulsation of the temporal vessels may be greater on the affected side and distended veins may be seen to arch across the forehead or temple. Thickened vessels may be visible in temporal arteritis.

The head may be held to one side, with the neck rotated, in some cases of posterior fossa tumour, resembling spasmodic torticollis in posture.

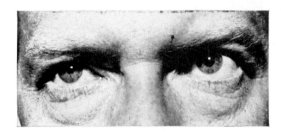

Figure 5.1. Paralysis of the ocular sympathetic nerve during an attack of cluster headache. The conjunctiva is injected on the affected side and a tear can be seen glistening in the conjunctival sac

Mental State

The mental state of the patient will have been assessed superficially during history-taking. Drowsiness, confusion or disorientation may indicate a space-occupying lesion or diffuse cerebral disorder such as meningitis or encephalitis. There may be indications of a focal cortical lesion preventing normal appreciation of the body image or understanding of the written or spoken word, which might thus give a false impression of general intellectual deterioration. The patient may be unable to express himself in words, mime, or writing, or to calculate or perform routine tasks, or distinguish between right and left because of a lesion of the dominant hemisphere. If cortical function is intact, the emotional tone of the patient must be assessed and a state of agitation or depression recognized.

Speech

If the patient is dysphasic, a note must always be made as to whether he or she is right or left handed. The left hemisphere is almost invariably responsible for speech mechanisms in right-handed patients, but in left-handers dysphasia may result from lesions in either hemisphere.

Skull

The skull must always be examined in patients with headache. This may seem self-evident but is often forgotten. A search of the scalp may disclose local infection, bone tumour or the hardened tender arteries of temporal arteritis (*see Figure 7.1*). The bones may be sensitive to percussion overlying inflamed sinuses or mastoid processes. The fontanelles should be palpated in infants since bulging of the fontanelles is a direct indication of increased intracranial pressure. It is worthwhile measuring the head circumference in a child at its widest point since repeated measurements are of value in detecting progressive hydrocephalus.

A short neck makes one think of congenital platybasia which may cause a slowly progressive hydrocephalus.

Auscultation of the skull (listening over the orbits, temples and mastoid processes) may disclose a systolic bruit in the case of aneurysm, angioma, vascular tumours or stenosis of the cranial vessels. When the examiner is listening over the closed eyelids, the patient is requested to open the other eye and hold the breath to prevent eyelid flutter and breath sounds from obscuring a bruit. Skull bruits are often normal in children under the age of 10 years and may be discounted unless loud and unilateral. An unexpected dividend from auscultation of the skull is that the sound of muscle contraction may be heard over the temporal and frontal muscles in patients who are unable to relax. Detecting this constant noise of muscle fibres straining one against the other makes one aware of nervous tension which might previously have been concealed.

Spine

The cervical spine is tested for tenderness and mobility. Resistance of the neck to passive flexion and Kernig's sign are usually present in meningeal irritation.

Gait and Stance

An unsteady wide-based gait may be observed as a result of cerebellar disturbance. It may indeed be the only sign of a midline cerebellar lesion in the early stages. The author recalls a one-legged man who suddenly lost the ability to walk with a crutch. There was no evidence of a cerebellar lesion other than his one-legged ataxia. Subsequent events disclosed a secondary carcinoma from the lung in the vermis of the cerebellum.

Special Senses

Smell

The nostrils are often blocked in rhinitis and sinusitis so that the sense of smell cannot be adequately assessed. The sense of smell may be lost when the olfactory nerve is damaged by head injury or

29

by a tumour in the vicinity of the olfactory groove. The sense of smell should always be tested when a patient's intellectual ability has deteriorated since a fronto-temporal tumour may cause both anosmia and mental confusion.

Vision

Circumcorneal injection may be observed in acute glaucoma and increased intra-ocular pressure may give rise to a palpable firmness of the eye. The significance of changes in visual acuity, visual fields and optic fundi is too large a subject to be encompassed here. It is sufficient to say that the visual fields of every patient complaining of a headache which does not conform to a typical benign pattern should be tested to confrontation and the optic fundi should always be examined.

The most common question to be decided is the presence or absence of papilloedema. Swelling of the optic disc usually starts at the poles and spreads to the nasal aspect of the disc before the temporal margin. The optic cup becomes filled-in and pulsation of veins where they cross over the rim of the optic cup can no longer be seen. If, after careful examination by an ophthalmologist, there is any dispute about whether an unusual appearance of the optic discs could be one of the forms of congenital pseudopapilloedema, the matter can be settled by fundus photography after the injection of fluorescein.

Swelling of the optic disc in optic (retrobulbar) neuritis is called papillitis and the appearance may be indistinguishable from papilloedema. Unlike papilloedema, papillitis causes severe impairment of vision. There is only slight restriction of the peripheral visual fields in papilloedema and the blind spot enlarges as swelling of the disc increases, since the blind spot is the projection of the optic disc in the visual fields.

Optic atrophy may result from interference with the blood supply to the optic nerve, long-standing papilloedema, retrobulbar neuritis or compression of the optic nerve or the optic chiasm. Occasionally a lesion behind the eye such as meningioma growing from the sphenoid wing compresses one optic nerve and its surrounding subarachnoid space, and then expands sufficiently to increase intra-cranial pressure or to impair venous return from the other eye so that papilloedema develops on the side opposite to the origin of the lesion. This combination of optic atrophy in one eye and papilloedema in the other is known as the Foster Kennedy syndrome.

Subhyaloid haemorrhages may be observed after subarachnoid bleeding, and perivascular nodules may rarely be seen in tuberculous meningitis or disseminated lupus erythematosus. Circumscribed areas of choroidal atrophy may be a sign of toxoplasmosis.

Hearing

The eardrums should be inspected, particularly in children, since otitis media may spread centrally to cause thrombosis of the lateral sinus (otitic hydrocephalus) or to form an abscess of temporal lobe or cerebellum. Conduction deafness is demonstrated by tuning fork tests in the case of otitis media or Eustachian catarrh. A unilateral nerve deafness should be further investigated by audiometry, loudness balance tests, caloric responses, radiography of the petrous temporal bone, and possibly tomography or posterior fossa myelography, to ensure that an acoustic neurinoma is not missed.

Other Cranial Nerves

A latent ocular imbalance may be unmasked by any infectious or debilitating illness and give rise to diplopia which may be misinterpreted as indicating a paresis of one or other of the extraocular muscles. A sixth nerve palsy may be found on the side of a lateral sinus thrombosis, and bilateral sixth nerve palsies may be found with any case of acute hydrocephalus or cerebral oedema because the sixth nerves are compressed in their long intracranial course by the expanded brain.

Progressive enlargement of the pupil on one side, with or without other signs of a third nerve palsy, is an indication for immediate action since the third nerve may be compressed by any expanding lesion forcing the uncus and medial aspect of the temporal lobe downwards through the tentorial opening into the posterior fossa. It can be taken as a rule that the dilated pupil is always on the side of the expanding lesion (such as a subdural haematoma) and exceptions to this rule are rare indeed. Inability to elevate both eyes is a sign of compression of the midbrain (Parinaud's syndrome) but it should be remembered that many elderly patients have difficulty in elevating the eyes.

The sudden onset of a third nerve palsy with pain behind the eye is most frequently caused by the sudden enlargement of an aneurysm (*see Figure 6.1*), although this may also occur in the rare syndrome of ophthalmoplegic migraine.

If the patient's consciousness becomes impaired so that voluntary eye movements are no longer possible, the integrity of the third, fourth and sixth nerves may be tested by the 'doll's eyes manoeuvre'. When the head is rotated to one side, the eyes roll to the opposite

31

side, thus producing the movements of lateral conjugate deviation. Similarly, if the chin is pushed down on the chest the eyes elevate and if the head is extended the eyes roll downwards.

The presence of Horner's syndrome in cluster headache has already been mentioned, and it may also be seen occasionally in migraine. The pupil of one side may remain small between paroxysms of cluster headache or after a severe attack of migraine. Both pupils may be small in a pontine lesion.

Any cranial nerve may be involved by direct compression. It is particularly important to test facial sensation carefully, including 2-point discrimination on the lip, and to check the corneal responses in patients with trigeminal neuralgia. If there is any sensory deficit the patient must be suspected of having a lesion compressing the trigeminal nerve or a pontine plaque of multiple sclerosis.

If corticobulbar pathways are involved, weakness of the lower face will be detected and the jaw jerk and facial reflexes may increase. A bifrontal lesion will result in a pouting of the lips on tapping in the midline between the nose and mouth.

Motor System

Signs of an upper motor neurone or cerebellar disturbance may be detected with an expanding intracranial lesion. When the patient's arms are extended and the eyes are closed, the arm may slowly fall away on the affected side. With an upper motor neurone (pyramidal) lesion, muscle tone may be increased and movements of the fingers become slow and clumsy. Power is reduced, particularly in the extensor and abductor groups of the upper limbs and flexors of the lower limbs. This distribution of weakness is characteristic of an upper motor neurone lesion, whether or not the deep reflexes are increased or the plantar response is extensor on that side.

A hemiparesis is most commonly found on the side opposite to a cerebral lesion but in a minority of patients with a rapidly expanding mass, such as subdural haematoma, the hemiparesis is found on the same side as the lesion. The reason for this is that the growing mass pushes the midbrain over on to the tentorial edge so that the opposite cerebral peduncle is compressed. Since the pyramidal tracts cross below this level, the hemiparesis is on the same side as the causative lesion. Bilateral upper motor neurone signs may result from midbrain compression. A grasp reflex indicates a lesion of the opposite frontal lobe. An interesting sign, known as the palmar-mental response, may be elicited in patients with frontal lobe lesions. Stroking the thenar eminence firmly evokes a brief contraction of the muscles of the chin on the same side.

With a cerebellar lesion, the affected side is hypotonic. When the elbows are resting on a table with forearms vertical and wrist muscles relaxed, the hand hangs lower on the affected side. If the eyes are closed and the arms are lifted suddenly to a point at right angles to the body the arm on the affected side overshoots and oscillates. The knee jerk is pendular on the affected side. Rapid and alternating movements are impaired and finger–nose and heel–shin co-ordination is defective. The gait is wide-based and halting, and the patient turns jerkily 'by numbers' and tends to stumble to the side of the lesion.

Sensory System

A parietal lobe disturbance may cause subtle sensory deficit with difficulty in discriminating two points or recognizing objects placed in the hand. Long sensory tracts may be involved with deeply-placed cerebral lesions or brain stem disorders, resulting in a more clear-cut sensory disturbance.

Sphincters and Sexual Functions

Urgency of micturition may appear with upper motor neurone lesions, and a casual approach towards the time and place of relaxing the sphincters may be a feature of frontal lobe disturbance. Impotence can result from a temporal lobe lesion. The author recently saw a woman with a frontal lobe tumour present with urinary incontinence while her intellect was sufficiently preserved for her to be distressed by the trail she left behind her.

General Examination

The presence of brownish patches in the skin (*café au lait* patches), with or without cutaneous neurofibromas (*Figure 5.2*) indicates that the patient has a greater chance than the average of harbouring an intracranial tumour or phaeochromocytoma. Not only neurofibromas but also meningiomas and gliomas are more common in neurofibromatosis or its formes frustes. The observation of cutaneous angiomas raises the possibility of an intracerebral angioma. Peutz–Jeghers syndrome is an unusual familial condition characterized by dark pigmentation on the lips and buccal mucosa which is associated with polyposis of the small intestine. There may be an increased tendency to intracranial tumour in this condition as there is in polyposis coli, since I have seen such a patient with multiple intracranial meningiomas.

33

D

Smoothness of the skin, paucity of body hair and testicular atrophy should be looked for as signs of pituitary deficiency.

Any scar in the skin warrants an enquiry about the nature of the lesion removed, as melanoma is notorious for presenting with metastases in the nervous system years after the primary tumour has been removed. Skin rashes are of importance in many infectious processes, such as meningococcaemia, glandular fever and the exanthemata, associated with headache.

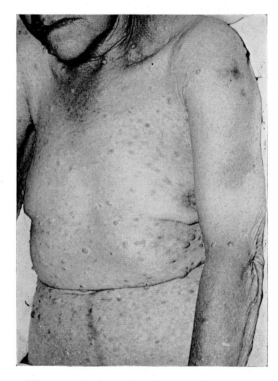

Figure 5.2. Neurofibromatosis, a condition associated with an increased incidence of acoustic neurinoma and other intracranial tumours. The skin lesions are usually soft to palpation

The association of a thin build with long fingers and toes and a high arched palate, known as Marfan's syndrome, carries an increased liability to intracranial aneuryms. Other inconstant features include hypertension from coarctation of the aorta, congenital heart defects and congenital dislocation of the lenses of the eye, which transmits a noticeable quivering movement to the iris on sudden eye movements.

Enlargement of lymph glands and spleen is related to the problem of headache in glandular fever, blood dyscrasias and the reticuloses.

Ecchymoses and purpura may be observed in thrombocytopenic purpura with neurological complications.

Urine testing does not contribute to the solution of most headache problems but the presence of albuminuria may be relevant to some causes of headache. The finding of a cardiac valvular defect should suggest the possibility of cerebral emboli (from atrial clot or subacute bacterial endocarditis) where transient cerebral episodes and headache are of recent onset.

Since most systemic disorders may have a neurological component, and most cerebral disorders may have headache as a symptom, there is no need to catalogue all the possible signs which could be be unearthed by careful examination which may bear direct relevance to the problem of headache. Having said this, it must be added that the majority of patients complaining of chronic headache do not have physical signs which pertain to their main symptom, unless we include constant muscular overactivity, the inability to relax, which is dealt with elsewhere. A number of other minor problems which require attention may be disclosed by a careful examination; many of them may have been a source of worry to the patient although unmentioned in the original history. There is no better start to the reassurance of a patient than the knowledge that a proper physical examination has been carried out as part of a careful clinical assessment.

6—Intracranial Sources of Headache

And he said unto his father, my head, my head. And he said to a lad, carry him to his mother. And when he had taken him, and brought him to his mother, he sat on her knees till noon, and then died.

(2 Kings IV, 19–20.)

Walton[202] suggests that this may be an early recorded case of subarachnoid haemorrhage. If so, the unusual sequel is worth noting. The prophet Elisha was summoned and as he was approaching he was met with the news that 'there was neither voice, nor hearing . . . . the child is not awaked'. Elisha 'went up and lay upon the child, and put his mouth upon his mouth . . . . and the flesh of the child waxed warm . . . . The child sneezed seven times, and the child opened his eyes'.

The sudden onset of headache, followed by loss of consciousness with recovery after resuscitation, makes a dramatic early description of headache of intracranial origin whether the cause was subarachnoid haemorrhage, as Walton suggests, or another intracranial disorder such as encephalitis.

MENINGEAL IRRITATION

The presence of blood in the subarachnoid space causes an inflammatory response in the meninges, probably because of the release of chemical agents.[100] Heparinized whole blood does not produce pain when applied to a blister base, unless it has been retained in a syringe for several minutes. In these circumstances platelets break down and release serotonin, and the plasma kinin-forming system is activated. The pain of injury or inflammation, as well as the pain provoked by extravascular blood, appears to be caused by the concerted action of substances which are contained in whole blood and are formed from inactive plasma precursors. Serotonin and kinins are probably the most important in this respect.

The chemical excitation of nerve endings in the meninges produces a reflex spasm of the neck extensors and sometimes of the lumbar muscles, which is analogous to the contraction of the abdominal wall resulting from peritoneal inflammation, and known as muscle 'guarding'. Muscle spasm consequent upon meningeal irritation gives rise to the physical signs of neck rigidity and Kernig's sign.

Subarachnoid Haemorrhage

Bleeding into the subarachnoid space may take place after head injury, or secondary to an intracerebral haemorrhage or 'spontaneously' in patients with cerebral aneurysm or angioma. Less commonly, bleeding may be the result of blood dyscrasias, haemorrhage from cerebral tumour, or some form of arteritis. The ratio of aneurysm to angioma as a cause of subarachnoid haemorrhage varies in different Western series from 5:1 to 25:1. The pattern is quite different in Asia, where angioma is more common. The headache of subarachnoid haemorrhage follows exertion in about one-third of patients. It usually starts suddenly and dramatically, 'like a blow on the head'. There may be a poorly localized sensation of something giving way inside the head, followed by unilateral headache which rapidly becomes generalized and spreads to the back of the head and neck, accompanied by photophobia. The patient may lose consciousness, with or without an epileptic seizure. The neck is usually rigid, and focal neurological signs are found if the aneurysm has compressed cranial nerves in enlarging or has bled into the brain substance (*Figures 6.1 and 6.2*). Pain in the back and legs may follow a subarachnoid haemorrhage after some hours or days, because of blood irritating the lumbo-sacral nerve roots. Haemorrhages may be seen in the fundi, spreading out from the optic discs, in some 7 per cent of patients, and papilloedema is found in 13 per cent.[202] Fever, albuminuria, glycosuria, hypertension and electrocardiographic changes may be present in the acute phase.

The diagnosis is made clinically and confirmed by lumbar puncture, when uniformly blood-stained fluid is withdrawn. After 4–12 hours, xanthochromia of the cerebrospinal fluid becomes apparent and it disappears from 12 to 40 days after the haemorrhage. A lymphocytic cellular reaction and increase in CSF protein to 70–130 mg/100 ml usually follows subarachnoid haemorrhage.[202]

When the patient is conscious, it is best to arrange for transfer as soon as practicable to a neurological centre for cerebral angiography and surgical treatment should a suitable vascular malformation be demonstrated. If no aneurysm or angioma can be found, the patient is confined to bed for 4–6 weeks, and resumes normal activities gradually.

37

The Relationship of Aneurysm and Angioma to Migraine

Of 220 patients with arteriovenous malformations or angiomas diagnosed by carotid angiography at the National Hospital for Nervous Diseases, London, 12 (5 per cent) were found to have a history of migraine.[26] In Walton's series of 312 cases of subarachnoid haemorrhage, 16 (5 per cent) gave a definite history of migraine. Six of his patients lost their migraine attacks after the episode of haemorrhage. Davis found that 6 per cent of 431 patients presenting

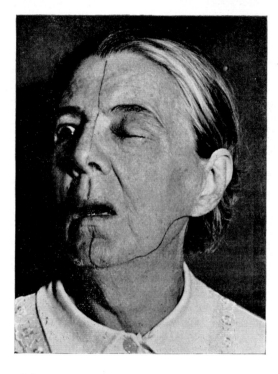

Figure 6.1. Loss of sensibility over the left half of the face with a complete left ptosis (third cranial nerve palsy). The onset was sudden with intense pain behind the left eye

with subarachnoid haemorrhage had a migrainous history.[56] The incidence of 5–6 per cent in these series is not very different from that of the general population. In contrast, Wolff found that 7 out of 46 patients with subarachnoid haemorrhage had suffered from migraine and another 12 had periodic recurrent headaches. However, the side of the aneurysm did not always relate to the side of the headache, and Wolff considered that the headache was independent of the presence or absence of aneurysm.[214] It remains uncertain from published statistics whether the association between migraine

38

and intracranial vascular malformations is more than could be expected by chance. Certainly carotid arteriography is not indicated solely because migraine attacks habitually affect the same side of the head. If the patient also has a loud intracranial bruit, or is subject to focal fits affecting the opposite side of the body, or has had a subarachnoid haemorrhage, then the likelihood of a positive result from carotid angiography is greatly increased. Some patients with cerebral angiomas have repeated small subarachnoid haemorrhages which are confused with migraine attacks or are thought to be episodes of 'encephalitis'.

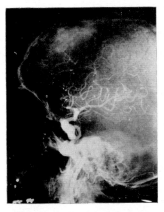

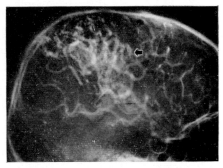

Figure 6.3. A large arteriovenous malformation demonstrated by carotid angiography in a young woman who suffered from classical migraine and repeated subarachnoid haemorrhages (case history in text)

Figure 6.2. Left carotid angiogram of the same patient as in Figure 6.1, showing a large aneurysm arising from the carotid siphon in a suitable position to compress the third cranial nerve and all three divisions of the trigeminal nerve

Case Report

The following is a case of cerebral angioma presenting as migraine with repeated subarachnoid haemorrhage.

A trained nurse aged 24 years had suffered from migraine headache since the age of 8 years. The attacks recurred about once a month and were always preceded by a sensation of 'pins and needles' spreading over the left side of the body. This sensation lasted for 10–30 minutes and was followed by a throbbing right-sided headache and nausea. The early administration of oral ergotamine tartrate aborted the majority of attacks. At the age of 13 years she had a particularly severe episode with neck stiffness and drowsiness which was thought to be a

39

viral meningoencephalitis. When aged 18 years she experienced a severe pain in the back of the neck followed by vomiting and neck stiffness. This pain eased but later she developed a severe right frontal headache with left-sided paraesthesiae which persisted for 2 hours. On examination her neck was rigid and a bruit was heard over both orbits, louder on the right side. A lumbar puncture disclosed uniformly blood-stained fluid and carotid angiography demonstrated an extensive intracerebral angioma (*Figure 6.3*). Since then she has been maintained on methysergide 1 mg three times daily and has been subject to three or four typical migraine headaches each year. There have been two more severe episodes with neck stiffness, one of which was proven by lumbar puncture to be a subarachnoid haemorrhage.

Meningitis and Encephalitis

The headache of intracranial inflammation may rarely present so acutely as to resemble subarachnoid haemorrhage, but more commonly the onset is gradual over hours or days. The pain is bilateral, extends down the neck, is associated with photophobia, and is made worse by head movement. The patient commonly has a fever and neck stiffness on examination.

The diagnosis is made by clinical assessment and lumbar puncture. The CSF contains an excess of cells, mostly neutrophils in pyogenic infections and in the acute phase of some cases of viral encephalitis. A purely lymphocytic pleocytosis usually indicates a viral infection but may be found in some cases of tuberculous or cryptococcal meningitis. A low CSF glucose value (in the absence of hypoglycaemia) means that the infecting organism is metabolizing glucose and indicates a pyogenic, tuberculous or torular infection. An exception to this rule is the unusual condition of meningitis carcinomatosa in which the meninges are infiltrated and ensheathed with malignant cells which multiply so rapidly that the CSF glucose level drops. The reticuloses and secondary melanoma may present in this way and the author has seen several cases of primary sarcoma of the meninges with a meningitic onset and multiple nerve root involvement.

Post-pneumoencephalographic Reaction

The introduction of air or oxygen into the subarachnoid space for diagnostic purposes (pneumoencephalography, air encephalography, air study) leads to a sterile inflammatory reaction which occasionally simulates meningoencephalitis in its severity. Samples of CSF taken during or after the air study often show a lymphocytic pleocytosis. In the more severe cases, the patient complains of photophobia and neck stiffness and may vomit so that the physician thinks of the possibility of meningitis induced by contamination at the time of lumbar puncture. The author has never seen this happen, whereas sterile reactions following pneumoencephalography are not uncommon. The inflammatory response is superimposed on the natural tendency to headache after lumbar puncture, caused by the lowered CSF pressure. The reaction is generally less in patients with large cerebral ventricles resulting from cerebral atrophy and is always greater when air passes over the surface of the cerebral hemispheres in the subarachnoid space. Some patients are free of headache the day after an air study but others continue to have headache for as long as 7–14 days after the procedure. Recent studies have shown that the introduction of methyl-prednisolone acetate 40 mg into the CSF at the conclusion of the air study reduces the frequency of unpleasant reactions. Apart from this the only therapeutic measures are to administer analgesics as required, to keep patients lying flat in bed and encourage them to drink a lot of fluid until the headache subsides.

TRACTION ON, OR DISPLACEMENT OF, INTRACRANIAL VESSELS

Space-Occupying Lesions

Unless a tumour or other space-taking lesion occupies a strategic position along the line of the drainage pathways of the cerebral ventricles, it is able to reach a considerable size before causing headache. Since the intracranial vessels have to be pushed aside before pain is registered, infiltrating tumours such as the gliomas may extend throughout one hemisphere without causing headache, because the position of large vessels may remain undisturbed until the last stages of the disease. Tumours which compress the brain from outside, such as meningiomas, are likely to cause fits, focal cerebral symptoms, progressive impairment of intellectual function or other neurological deficit before they produce headache.

Subdural haematoma, on the other hand, advances on a wide front so that a large surface area of brain is forced inwards and downwards (*Figure 6.4*). It almost invariably presents with headache, usually accompanied by drowsiness, and must be suspected in any patient of any age in whom these symptoms have progressed steadily over some days or weeks, even in the absence of a history of head injury. When the condition is well advanced, the patient usually develops a hemiparesis on the side opposite the subdural haematoma.

Occasionally the hemiparesis is on the same side as the lesion because the midbrain has been displaced by the expanding mass so that the opposite cerebral peduncle impinges on the tentorium. The author has seen in some patients a bilateral spastic weakness of the limbs. The third nerve, which crosses from midbrain to the cavernous sinus, is stretched as the enlarging mass forces part of the temporal lobe down through the tentorial opening on that side. Signs of a third nerve palsy (ptosis, enlarged pupil, failure of the eye to adduct or elevate fully) are therefore indications for immediate action because midbrain compression and irreversible damage are not far away.

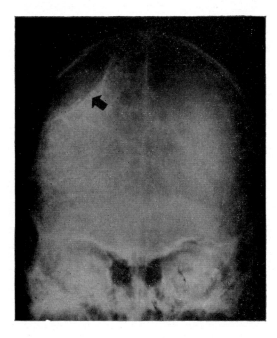

Figure 6.4. The capillary phase of a carotid angiogram outlining a convex filling defect characteristic of subdural haematoma

Case Report

The following is a case of subdural haematoma with quadriparesis resulting from a trivial injury.

A woman aged 48 years was holidaying in Noumea when she became aware of a right frontal headache which was worse on sudden movement of the head. The pain became worse over 12 days so that she returned to Sydney. She was drowsy but able to give a clear history, and could not recollect any head injury in the past 2 years. On examination of the fundi, the optic cups were indistinct and there was no venous pulsation. There was an incomplete third nerve palsy on the right. Flexor groups

42

were weak in both lower limbs, with increased deep reflexes and extensor plantar responses. Immediate carotid angiography disclosed a large right subdural haematoma which was removed later that evening. When she had recovered her normal mental acuity she recalled that 6 weeks previously she had stood up suddenly in the kitchen, banging her head on an open cupboard door, which made her 'see stars' for a moment.

Increased Intracranial Pressure

Any lesion which obstructs the flow of CSF from the lateral ventricles through the foramen of Monro, third ventricle, aqueduct, fourth ventricle and its exit foramina, or prevents the passage of CSF over the cortex to its absorption site (*Figure 6.5*), will cause a rapid increase in intracranial pressure so that headache becomes the main presenting symptom.

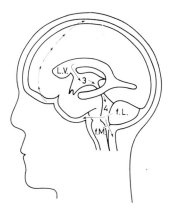

Figure 6.5. Diagram of the circulation of the cerebrospinal fluid from its origin in the choroid plexus, through the ventricular system to its absorption from the arachnoid villi of the superior sagittal sinus, after its passage in the subarachnoid space over the cerebral hemispheres. Obstruction at any point of the conducting system may increase intracranial pressure and lead to hydrocephalus. L.V. = lateral ventricle. 3, 4 = third and fourth ventricle respectively. F.L. = foramen of Luschka. F.M. = foramen of Magendie

M 71 / 107 (6·5)

A tumour in the vicinity of the third ventricle may also interfere intermittently with the function of the midbrain reticular formation so that posture cannot be maintained and the patient thus suffers from 'drop attacks,' in which he or she slumps heavily to the ground.

Case Report

The following is a case of colloid cyst of the third ventricle presenting with headache, myoclonus and drop attacks.

A bank officer aged 36 complained of bilateral headache for the past 6 years, which extended down the neck and usually recurred every day, although there had been breaks of up to one week without headache. The pain was brought on by standing suddenly and lasted from 1 hour to the whole day. It was associated with slight blurring of the periphery of both visual fields and often with the 'jim-jams'. The 'jim-jams' either occurred on their own for 5–10 minutes, usually around noon, or preceded a headache. They consisted of trembling and weakness of the arms and legs, which caused him to drop things, and at times his legs buckled so that he had to support himself with his arms. On one occasion he lost consciousness suddenly without warning. He had always been a worrier, had lost four children at birth or shortly afterwards from Rh incompatibility and thought that he was becoming

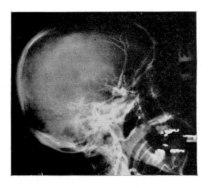

Figure 6.6. The presence of internal hydrocephalus may be detected by carotid angiography. The anterior cerebral artery is straightened and bowed upwards because of enlargement of the lateral ventricles. The middle cerebral artery is similarly displaced by the dilated temporal horn

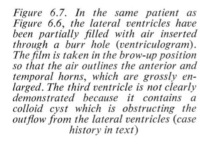

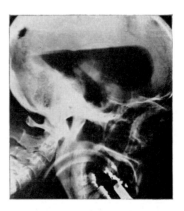

Figure 6.7. In the same patient as Figure 6.6, the lateral ventricles have been partially filled with air inserted through a burr hole (ventriculogram). The film is taken in the brow-up position so that the air outlines the anterior and temporal horns, which are grossly enlarged. The third ventricle is not clearly demonstrated because it contains a colloid cyst which is obstructing the outflow from the lateral ventricles (case history in text)

depressed like his mother who had recently been treated by electro-convulsive therapy. Physical examination and an electroencephalogram were normal. He did not report again for 12 months, at which time he had been confused and drowsy for 2 weeks. He was found to have bilateral papilloedema, a left grasp reflex and extensor plantar responses. Carotid angiography (*Figure 6.6*) and ventriculography (*Figure 6.7*) revealed an internal hydrocephalus caused by tumour of the third ventricle. A colloid cyst was removed through the foramen of Monro. After 1 week of akinetic mutism the patient recovered well and returned to work after some months although his memory remained impaired.

44

Stenosis of the aqueduct leading from the third ventricle to the fourth may be a congenital malformation which does not produce any symptoms until some systemic infection causes proliferation of its ependymal lining which then blocks the canal and produces an acute internal hydrocephalus.[161] Some cases of aqueduct stenosis may be caused by viral infections. Johnson and his colleagues showed that antibodies to mumps virus selectively accumulated in ependymal cells lining the aqueduct of suckling hamsters and that aqueduct stenosis consistently followed the innoculation of mumps virus although the infection was not apparent clinically.[99]

The aqueduct may also be obstructed by tumours in the vicinity of the midbrain.

Posterior Fossa Lesions

The aqueduct and fourth ventricle may be displaced or blocked by tumours of the posterior fossa. It is remarkable that tumours may grow to considerable size in the confined space of the posterior fossa without producing much in the way of symptoms or signs. The author has seen children and adults with large cystic astrocytomas and haemangioblastomas of the cerebellum whose only symptom apart from headache was unsteadiness of gait. There is no point in giving details here of the various types of posterior fossa tumours and the ways in which they may present. A unilateral nerve deafness warrants full investigation whether or not there are any other neurological symptoms because eighth nerve tumour should be diagnosed at an early stage, years before it is in a position to cause headache. Diplopia, facial paraesthesiae or pain, vertigo, ataxia, or any disturbance of speech or swallowing mechanisms obviously warrant investigation as soon as such symptoms appear.

A posterior fossa tumour may cause pain by direct compression of the fifth, seventh, ninth or tenth cranial nerves which may refer pain to the face, ear or throat. Pain is experienced in the neck because of irritation of the dura which is supplied by the upper three cervical nerve roots and reflex spasm of neck muscles may cause the head to be held to one side. Pain may also be referred to the eye and forehead by convergence of impulses from the upper cervical nerve roots upon neurones of the cervical cord which also serve the trigeminal pathways.[99] Finally, a generalized headache may be caused by blockage of the flow of CSF with resulting increase in intracranial pressure. Some of these points are illustrated by the following protocol.

Case Report

The following is a case of posterior fossa meningioma presenting with pain in the neck.

A woman aged 53 years noticed that her neck felt stiff when she looked up to hang clothes on a line, and ached when she was overtired. Since there was radiographic evidence of cervical disc degeneration, she was treated by cervical traction and manipulation which made the pain a little worse. One year later she began to be awakened from sleep at 2–3 a.m. about once a week by a bilateral headache which lasted for an hour. Neck pain persisted and, after another year had passed, occipital and frontal headaches were recurring daily. She then noticed a continuous dull ache in the left side of her face associated with a feeling of numbness involving the roof of her mouth on the left, which gradually crept over the cheek and the forehead. She felt nauseated and vomited without reason, which was attributed by the patient to nervous tension. The pain in her neck and back of the head became more severe and was particularly unpleasant after jolting or driving in a car. She noticed that she had to swallow twice to get food down, even after chewing it carefully, and she was a little unsteady on her feet at times.

On examination the optic fundi were normal. The left corneal reflex was depressed and 2-point discrimination was impaired on the left upper lip. Fine movements of the left arm and leg were a little clumsier than one would expect but there were no frank cerebellar signs. Carotid and vertebral angiography disclosed an internal hydrocephalus with a tumour circulation in the posterior fossa. On posturing the patient for posterior fossa craniotomy, the cardiac rhythm and respiration became irregular and remained so until the occipital bone was removed. A pressure cone of cerebellum was then seen to extend some 5 cm down the spinal canal to the third cervical vertebra. After removal of the posterior arch of the atlas and the spine and laminae of the second cervical vertebra, heartrate and respiration returned to normal. A large meningioma, approximately 4 cm in diameter was found to be compressing the cerebellum and cranial nerves and extending through the tentorium. It was satisfactorily removed, and another operation two months later was required to remove its equally large supratentorial extension. The patient recovered well and slowly resumed her usual activities. She remains well 2 years after operation.

A haemorrhage into the cerebellum can rapidly prove fatal if not recognized and treated surgically, because it rapidly compresses respiratory and vasomotor centres in the brainstem. The condition may readily be confused with vertebrobasilar insufficiency or thrombosis because it is liable to occur in the middle-aged or elderly hypertensive patient and presents with sudden severe occipital headache, vertigo, ataxia and vomiting. Nystagmus or deviation of the visual axes may be found on examination (*Figure 6.8*), together with incoordination of upper and lower limbs and ataxia. The patient usually becomes stuporose or unconscious so that the diagnosis may have to be made on the history of the onset. Posterior fossa craniotomy is the only measure which will prevent the patient's death. Like intracerebellar haemorrhage, a subdural haematoma in the posterior fossa is uncommon, but it is worth mentioning because it is a remediable condition which must be thought of before it can be diagnosed.

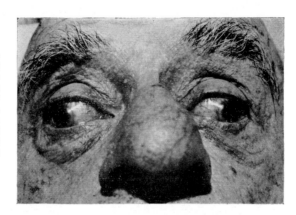

Figure 6.8. Deviation of the visual axes in an elderly patient with an acute intracerebellar haematoma, which was successfully removed. The patient recovered well but was left with severe ataxia of gait

Hydrocephalus may progress slowly from conditions in the region of the cisterna magna and foramen magnum. Tumours in this area, a congenital malformation known as the Dandy–Walker syndrome, and platybasia may be responsible for obstruction of the flow of CSF. Platybasia is a flattening of the floor of the posterior fossa with rotation of the anterior parts of the atlas and axis upwards so that a line drawn through the body of the atlas forms an angle of more than 13 degrees with the line of the hard palate[33] (*Figure 6.9*). It may be a congenital anomaly, often associated with spina bifida, or may develop through softening of the base of the skull in Paget's disease, osteoporosis or osteomalacia.

Communicating Hydrocephalus

The conditions so far considered produce an internal hydrocephalus with dilatation of the ventricular system on the central side of the block. Less commonly, the fluid may emerge freely from the fourth ventricle by the foramina of Magendie and Luschka but be impeded from ascending through the basal cisterns and subarachnoid space because of adhesive arachnoiditis. It has long been recognized that this may be a cause of hydrocephalus in tuberculous or other meningitis, but only recently it has been shown that the condition may develop quietly in the older patient, causing dementia.[5] Progressive arachnoiditis may follow head injury or subarachnoid haemorrhage, or arise without obvious reason. The condition is

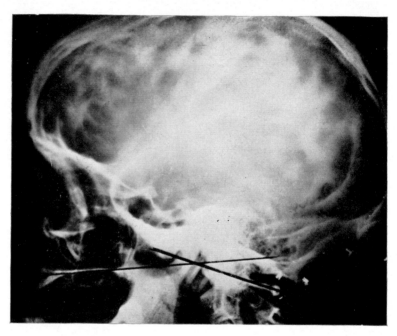

Figure 6.9. Radiological signs of long-standing hydrocephalus in a patient with congenital platybasia. The skull has a 'beaten-copper' appearance ('thumbing' of the vault), and the posterior clinoid processes are decalcified by pressure from the dilated third ventricle. The lines drawn through the body of the atlas and in the plane of the hard palate intersect at an angle of more than 13 degrees, one of the criteria for the diagnosis of platybasia

suspected if pneumoencephalography demonstrates a large ventricular system, without the pooling of air in the cortical sulci which is pathognomonic of cerebral atrophy. No matter how the head is manoeuvred, no air enters the subarachnoid space over the cerebral hemispheres. The diagnosis is confirmed by brain scanning after the insertion of a radioactive isotope into the CSF to determine its rate of clearance from the ventricular system. Like other forms of hydrocephalus the condition may improve following insertion into the lateral ventricle of a catheter, which is then run under the skin of

48

scalp and neck to be inserted through the jugular vein into the right atrium. The CSF thus drains into the venous circulation and a plastic valve prevents blood from passing into the CSF should the venous pressure become elevated.

Venous Sinus Thrombosis and Otitic Hydrocephalus

The lateral sinus may thrombose following infection of the middle ear and mastoid bone, causing cerebral oedema, termed 'otitic hydrocephalus'. There is no internal hydrocephalus since the ventricles are normal or small in size. The patient, usually a child, develops headache and papilloedema after an ear infection. The sixth nerve may be paralysed on the side of the lesion, or on both sides because of the nerves being stretched by the expanded brain. Radiographs commonly show opacity of the mastoid air cells. Treatment is directed to the infected ear and mastoid (which may include mastoidectomy and removal of clot from the lateral sinus) and, by the measures described below, to reducing cerebral oedema.

Case Report

The following is the report of a case of 'otitic hydrocephalus' with bilateral sixth nerve palsy.

A boy aged 4 years developed a typical attack of measles. Nine days after the disappearance of the rash he awoke during the night with pain in the right ear, and vomited. He was treated with tetracycline but complained of headache and noises in the head for the next 24 hours. He was admitted to hospital because of further vomiting and a slight increase in temperature. His fundi were normal, his right ear drum was reddened and there was slight neck stiffness. A lumbar puncture disclosed that his CSF was completely normal. He continued to have a mild fever and bilateral headache and developed a loose cough with occasional vomiting. Antibiotic treatment was altered to penicillin and then to ampicillin. One week after the onset of pain in the right ear, he was found to have a bilateral sixth nerve palsy and papilloedema. Radiographs of the skull showed opacity of the mastoid air cells on the right side. Ventriculography demonstrated that the lateral ventricles were smaller than normal. He recovered rapidly following ventricular drainage and mastoidectomy. Frusemide was used to reduce intracranial pressure after the ventricular drain was removed, and lumbar puncture confirmed the effectiveness of this treatment.

Raised Venous Pressure

Mediastinal obstruction and emphysema are said to increase venous pressure sufficiently to interfere with cerebral venous drainage and cause papilloedema. Hypoxia associated with these conditions probably increases the tendency to oedema of the brain and optic nerve.

Cerebral Oedema from Other Causes

A sudden elevation of the blood pressure, as in malignant hypertension, may cause headache, presumably through the mechanism of cerebral oedema displacing pain-sensitive blood vessels, since the headache is relieved by the intravenous infusion of hypertonic solutions such as 50 per cent glucose but not when CSF pressure is reduced by lumbar puncture.[214] One hemisphere may swell following infarction, as a result of thrombosis of the internal carotid artery, or thrombosis or embolism of one of its main branches. Headache is commonly a symptom of cerebral infarction. Cerebral oedema may be sufficiently pronounced to cause papilloedema after internal carotid thrombosis, thus simulating an acute presentation of cerebral tumour.

The syndrome of *benign intracranial hypertension*[70] may be encountered in children given large doses of vitamin A, and in males following head injury. It may appear spontaneously in fat young women, in women during pregnancy, or in women taking hormonal preparations to avoid pregnancy. It has been reported as an idiosyncratic reaction to certain drugs such as nalidixic acid and the tetracyclines. The patient presents with headache and papilloedema. The CSF pressure is elevated but investigations exclude the presence of a space-occupying lesion or obstructive hydrocephalus. The ventricles are small because of cerebral oedema. The condition may subside without specific treatment, but repeated lumbar puncture, a potent diuretic such as frusemide, or high dosage with adrenal corticosteroids (dexamethasone 32–64 mg daily) may be required to reduce cerebral oedema and prevent optic atrophy.

Hypocalcaemia may produce cerebral oedema, papilloedema and fits. Prolonged dosage with corticosteroids has been reported as causing headache, vomiting, papilloedema, diplopia and drowsiness.[60] Addison's disease may also be responsible for cerebral oedema and papilloedema.[98]

Case Report

The following is the report of a case of Addisonian crisis with meningeal irritation and papilloedema, simulating meningoencephalitis.

A woman aged 32 years had her sixth child uneventfully but was unable to breast feed her baby for more than a few days, which was unusual for her. About 1 month later she developed headache, rigors and vomiting, which recovered without any treatment, although she continued to have slight bilateral headaches. Her husband noted that she was more irritable than usual and rather vague in her manner. Several weeks later she complained of a sore throat and awoke one night with severe headache, rigors and vomiting, and became drowsy. Her general practitioner gave her an intravenous injection of tetracycline and arranged for her transfer to Sydney by ambulance. When admitted to the hospital, she was stuporose, restless and irritable, curling up to avoid the light. She was moderately pigmented on exposed areas with a prominent linea nigra and dark nipples, but there was no buccal pigmentation. Her colouring was thought to be consistent with being a country dweller in a sunny climate, particularly as she had recently completed a pregnancy. Neck stiffness, Kernig's sign and early bilateral papilloedema were noted. Her blood pressure was 130/80 mmHg. On lumbar puncture, the flow of CSF was slow and the pressure could not be measured. The fluid contained 100 polymorphonuclear cells and 60 lymphocytes/mm^3, and a protein content of 80 mg/100 ml. Serum electrolytes were normal apart from sodium which was 130 mEq/litre. Radiographs of skull and chest and carotid arteriography were normal. She was thought to have a partly treated bacterial meningitis or viral meningoencephalitis, and penicillin, chloramphenicol and sulphadiazine were administered, although no organism was grown from CSF or blood cultures. Her temperature reached 39·5°C on several occasions and her blood pressure fell alarmingly to 80/50 mmHg. A repeated lumbar puncture showed that CSF pressure was 110 mm. The cellular and protein content was similar to that of the previous day and glucose content was 60 mg/100 ml. Corticosteroids were withheld because of the presumed infectious nature of the illness and she died that evening. Autopsy revealed that the brain was macroscopically and microscopically normal. There was a purulent pericarditis. The only adrenal tissue found was a sliver 2 mm thick on the right side which showed almost complete loss of adrenal cortex on histological examination.

Reduced Intracranial Pressure

The headache which often follows lumbar puncture is probably caused by continued leakage of CSF from the subarachnoid space after the procedure, which lowers intracranial pressure, withdrawing support for the brain, thus causing traction upon intracranial vessels. The frequency of such headaches may be reduced by using a fine-gauge needle, lying the patient on his front for 4 hours after lumbar puncture and maintaining bed rest for 24 hours afterwards. Should a headache ensue there is no treatment other than keeping the patient lying flat in bed, requesting him to drink as much fluid as possible and administering analgesics when required.

SIMPLE INTRACRANIAL VASODILATATION

The headache produced by histamine has been studied more than other forms of intracranial vascular headache and is considered in more detail in Chapters 9 and 10. Other vasodilators such as the nitrites will produce a similar headache. There is good evidence that such headaches are caused by distension of the arterial wall because they are reduced in intensity either by lowering the blood pressure or by increasing CSF pressure.[164] They are characteristically bilateral, throbbing in nature and made worse by jarring of the head or any sudden movement.

Intracranial vascular headache may be caused by head injury (post-concussional headache), circulating toxins in acute infectious febrile diseases and metabolic disturbances such as hypoxia, hypercapnia and hypoglycaemia. The headache which commonly follows an epileptic fit is probably the result of transient hypoxia and retention of carbon dioxide which are known to dilate cerebral vessels. The injection of foreign proteins, such as typhoid vaccine, produces fever and vascular headache. It is not certain whether 'hangover' headache is caused by breakdown products of alcohol acting as dilators of intracranial vessels, although the headache certainly has the clinical characteristics of an intracranial vascular headache. The use of monosodium glutamate in Chinese cuisine can produce a postprandial headache in the unwary gourmet. Hypoglycaemia may produce a vascular headache in some people who miss a regular meal-time, in those with carbohydrate intolerance, when headache appears several hours after meals, or in diabetic patients overdosed with insulin, patients with islet cell tumour or with endocrine disorders such as hypopituitarism and Addison's disease.[187] The diagnosis may be made by a 5-hour glucose tolerance test, blood glucose determination after a 48-hour fast, a tolbutamide tolerance test, plasma insulin levels, or a combination of these investigations.

Phenacetin and caffeine exert a vasoconstrictor effect on cranial vessels. It has been postulated that patients become habituated to headache preparations which contain them because a rebound headache occurs when their effect wears off after 3–4 hours.

The headache of cerebral vascular insufficiency is difficult to explain. It is known that thrombosis of one internal carotid artery may cause gross unilateral cerebral oedema with displacement of the intracranial vessels and headache of the affected side. However, headache may accompany transient episodes of insufficiency, commonly being felt in the frontal region when the internal carotid artery is affected and in the occipital region when the vertebro-basilar system is at fault.[69]. The mechanism of headache may be sudden dilatation of collateral channels in response to the sudden demand made upon them, but this is not known with certainty.

The headache of cerebral embolism is probably caused by cerebral oedema and the dilatation of collateral channels. *Figure 6.10* shows a mycotic aneurysm in a patient with subacute bacterial endocarditis who presented with left-sided headaches associated with transient aphasia and right hemiparesis. The diagnosis was complicated by a past history of migraine. Subacute bacterial endocarditis was confirmed by blood cultures but in spite of a satisfactory response

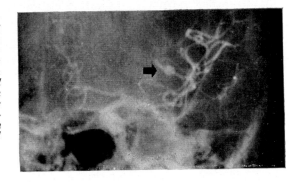

Figure 6.10. Mycotic aneurysm situated peripherally on a branch of the middle cerebral artery. The patient present with transient left-sided headaches, aphasia and right hemiparesis as the result of cerebral embolism from subacute bacterial endocarditis

to antibiotics, the patient developed intensely severe headache and died rapidly two weeks after the onset of her illness. At autopsy, the vegetations on the mitral valve were found to be healing satisfactorily. The left hemisphere was expanded by a large intra-cerebral haematoma.

A sudden increase in systemic blood pressure may cause headache, whether the circumstances be physiological, such as enthusiastic sexual intercourse, or pathological as with the hypertensive crises of phaeochromocytoma. The symptoms of phaeochromocytoma vary from patient to patient, one of the reasons being the proportion of adrenaline to noradrenaline produced by the tumour. Headache is commonly experienced in the early phase of the attack but may disappear when symptoms of blanching, sweating and tachycardia are well established, possibly because of the constriction of cranial vessels by circulating catecholamines. Pressor reactions have been reported when patients taking mono-amine oxidase (MAO) inhibitor drugs for depression or other reasons have drunk red wines and eaten cheese or other foods which are rich in tyramine. Noradrenaline is released by tyramine and cannot be catabolized because the activity of the responsible enzyme is suppressed. Similar adverse reactions may result from the combination of sympathomimetic drugs, such as ephedrine, imipramine, carbamazepine, and the amphetamines with MAO inhibitors. These hypertensive crises can be controlled by intravenous phentolamine.

There is evidence that migrainous subjects are more likely to develop hypertension in later life than the general population.[200] On the other hand, the onset of hypertension makes migraine worse in frequency and severity. Apart from the aggravation of pre-existing vascular headaches, there appears to be an association between hypertension and muscle-contraction headaches. There is still some doubt as to the frequency of a specific hypertensive headache which is present on awakening and settles down after some hours of activity. There are reports of headaches improving after the drug treatment of hypertension is initiated but the author has not seen any controlled observations. Wolff comments that the headache associated with hypertension often responds to rest or relaxation without substantial change in the level of blood pressure.[214]

EXERTIONAL AND COUGH HEADACHE

Hippocrates remarked that 'one should be able to recognize those who have headaches from gymnastic exercises, or running, or walking, or hunting, or any other unseasonable labour, or from immoderate venery'.[4] Headache caused by sexual intercourse or other forms of exertion is probably of intracranial origin in most instances, although some patients may describe throbbing and excessive pulsation in the temporal arteries. The author recalls two healthy young men who were subject to bilateral headaches on physical exertion. One was forced to stop playing cricket and the other was unable to dig in his garden for this reason. Both responded favourably to taking methysergide 2 mg the night before the projected exertion and repeating this dose in the morning. With this help, they were able to complete a day of cricket or gardening without headache although they remained aware of increased pulsation in the temples.

Sir Charles Symonds[190] described 27 patients with headache on coughing, 21 of whom did not have any demonstrable intracranial lesion. The recognition of 'benign cough headache' is of considerable importance. Once a tumour in the region of the foramen magnum or elsewhere interfering with the flow of cerebrospinal fluid through the ventricular system is excluded, the patient may be reassured. Of Symonds' 21 patients, 9 lost their headaches spontaneously and 6 improved with the course of time.

Rooke[160] considers that cough headache is a variety of exertional headache and recorded his experience with 103 patients who experienced transient headaches on running, bending, coughing, sneezing, lifting or straining at stool, in whom no intracranial disease could be detected, who were followed for 3 or more years. During the follow-up period, reinvestigation discovered structural lesions in 10 patients, such as Arnold–Chiari malformation, platybasia, subdural haematoma, and cerebral or cerebellar tumour. Of the remaining 93, 30 were free of headache within 5 years and 73 were improved or free of headache after 10 years. This type of headache was found in men more often than women in the ratio 4:1. The aetiology is unknown but Rooke observes that this form of headache may appear for the first time after a respiratory infection with cough and that some patients reported an abrupt recovery after the extraction of abscessed teeth, which had also been noted by Symonds.

7—Extracranial Sources of Headache, Psychogenic Pain, and Post-Traumatic Headache

Suppose a person to complain of pain upon the scalp, is it not very essential to know whether that pain is expressed by the fifth nerve or by the great or small occipital? Thus pain in the anterior and lateral part of the head, which are supplied by the fifth nerve, would suggest that the cause must be somewhere in the area of the distribution of the other portions of the fifth nerve. So if the pain be expressed behind, the cause must assuredly be connected with the great or small occipital nerve, and in all probability depends on disease of the spine between the first and second cervical vertebrae.

John Hilton (1805–1878)[91]

These remarks are part of the fourth lecture of a series of eighteen on 'Rest and Pain' given by Hilton between 1860 and 1862. They express admirably the approach to extracranial sources of headache, some of which are located in the skull or scalp, whereas others are referred from nearby areas, although not as often from the neck as Hilton implied. The most common types of extracranial headache are those caused by dilatation of the extracranial vessels, particularly migraine, and those caused by over-contraction of the muscles in the head and neck, muscle-contraction or tension headache. Migraine, cluster and tension headache present such difficulty in understanding and management that they warrant chapters to themselves. Certain variations on the theme of migraine, such as facial, ophthalmoplegic and hemiplegic migraine, are discussed as part of that disorder.

INFLAMMATION OF EXTRACRANIAL VESSELS

Collagen diseases such as polyarteritis nodosa and disseminated lupus erythematosus may affect the cranial vessels, but the author has never seen a patient with one of these disorders presenting with headache.

A related disease, *temporal or giant-cell arteritis,* usually presents with headache. It affects more patients of an older age group than the other collagen diseases, usually over the age of 55 years, although 1 patient aged 35 years has been reported. The superficial temporal arteries are not the only scalp vessels affected and the author examined one patient in whom all the scalp arteries were palpable as hard sinuous cords throughout their length on both sides of the head. The disorder may also involve intracranial vessels, particularly the ophthalmic artery, causing optic atrophy and blindness. The aorta, coronary, renal and iliac arteries have been implicated in some reported cases.

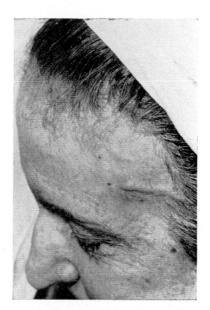

Figure 7.1. The characteristic appearance of temporal arteritis

Typical temporal arteritis starts with throbbing pain over the affected scalp arteries which become thickened and cease to pulsate (*Figure 7.1*). They are usually tender to the touch, and the skin may become red over the affected vessels. Vision is impaired in about one-half of the patients at some stage of the disease. Claudication of the muscles of mastication has been noticed by some patients. There may be associated symptoms caused by damage to intra-cranial vessels. Formed hallucinations have been described, including visions of flapping brightly coloured curtains, flowers, crowds of small children and menacing people, probably resulting from temporal lobe ischaemia.[87] Mental deterioration, vertigo and deafness, stroke and coronary thrombosis are other modes of presentation.

Symptoms of systemic disturbance, such as loss of weight, night sweats, aching of joints and muscles and a low grade fever are commonly associated,[147] thus merging into the syndrome known as 'polymyalgia rheumatica'.

Apart from obvious changes in the scalp vessels, the physical signs vary according to the extent of involvement of the cerebral and other arteries. The ophthalmoscopic picture of central retinal artery thrombosis may be seen, retinal ischaemia and oedema with dimpling in the macular region producing a greyish-red spot. At a later stage the optic disc becomes atrophic.

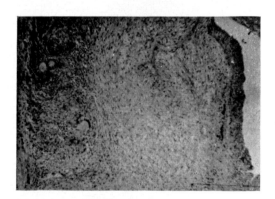

Figure 7.2. The biopsy of the vessel shown in Figure 7.1. The arterial wall is thickened with round cell infiltration and giant-cell formation

The erythrocyte sedimentation rate is greater than 45 mm/hr in the majority of patients and ranges up to 120 mm/hr. Electrophoresis of serum proteins demonstrates increase in alpha and beta globulin fractions. Most patients have a mild hypochromic anaemia and polymorphonuclear leucocytosis. Biopsy of the temporal artery (or the facial artery if this is more appropriate to the site of pain) shows thickening of the intima, fibrosis and cellular infiltration of the vessel wall, often with giant cells resembling those of tuberculous disease or sarcoidosis, and thrombus formation in the lumen (*see Figure 7.2*). The distribution of vascular changes may be patchy so that a negative biopsy does not necessarily negate the diagnosis. Arteriography of the external carotid circulation has recently been used to indicate the sites most severely involved so that an arterial biopsy may be selective.

The use of adrenal corticosteroids rapidly stops the pain and malaise of the syndrome and it is generally accepted that the risk of ophthalmic artery involvement is reduced to about half, but not completely obviated, by the use of steroids. Prednisone may be started in the dose of 40–60 mg daily and reduced slowly after some weeks to a maintenance dosage of 10–20 mg daily. Treatment may have to be continued for up to twelve months as relapse may take place if the patient is weaned off corticosteroids prematurely. Osteoporosis has to be guarded against in patients of this age group who are on longterm treatment and anabolic steroids, oestrogens or androgens may assist in its prevention. The E.S.R. and white cell count return to normal limits as the inflammation subsides with the use of steroids.

CRANIAL NERVE DISORDERS

Acute retrobulbar neuritis will be considered under the heading of pain referred from the eye.

Any lesion compressing the fifth, seventh, ninth or tenth cranial nerves can cause pain referred to the face, ear or throat, which may start with a jabbing neuralgic quality but soon develops an aching component persisting between the more severe paroxysms. Constant pain indicates that the condition is not one of idiopathic trigeminal or glossopharyngeal neuralgia. Impairment of sensation over the face, in the external auditory meatus or over the posterior pharyngeal wall supports the diagnosis of a focal abnormality in the posterior fossa. Sensory changes may be slight. A minor asymmetry of the corneal reflexes or defective discrimination of 2 points separated by 0·5 cm when touching the lips may be the only sign of trigeminal nerve deficit. A careful examination of the sensibility at the back of throat tested by prodding with a swab stick or long pin may reveal a slight diminution on one side. These signs warrant a full neurological investigation since tumour, aneurysm, abscess, osteomyelitis of the base of the skull and brainstem lesions such as multiple sclerosis may present in this way.

Trigeminal Neuralgia

Sensation is not lost in idiopathic trigeminal neuralgia (tic douloureux) or glossopharyngeal neuralgia and the pain remains true to a characteristic paroxysmal pattern. Kerr[103] listed the following characteristic features of trigeminal neuralgia.

(1) The onset is usually after the age of 40 years.
(2) Females are affected twice as often as males.

(3) The pain is present more often on the right side than the left in the ratio 3:2.

(4) The pain is limited strictly to some part of the distribution of the fifth cranial nerve. It usually starts in the second or third divisions, affecting cheek or chin. Less than 5 per cent start in the first division. About 3 per cent ultimately become bilateral.

(5) The quality of the pain is superficial, intense, brief and paroxysmal.

(6) Trigger points are present at some time in the course of the disease. The pain may be brought on by talking, chewing or swallowing or by touching the face or gums as in shaving or cleaning the teeth.

(7) There is a tendency to progression in the frequency and severity of episodes.

One might add to these points that the condition may have spontaneous remissions for months or years, and that pain of tic douloureux may be simulated by central as well as peripheral lesions. The incidence of trigeminal neuralgia in multiple sclerosis is 1–2 per cent. Looked at from the reverse direction, about 3 per cent of patients with trigeminal neuralgia have multiple sclerosis.[133] The syndrome differs from the idiopathic form only in that it usually occurs at a younger age, is more often bilateral, and lacks 'trigger areas'.

The aetiology of trigeminal neuralgia is uncertain. It may be a primary degenerative disease of the nerve or be caused by mechanical factors. It has been postulated that the internal carotid artery which lies directly beneath the trigeminal ganglion and adjacent posterior rootlets, may impinge on the second and third divisions at this point, since the bony roof of the carotid canal is often replaced by a thin layer of connective tissue.[103] Compression of the nerve could account for the breakdown of myelin sheaths in older patients. Demyelination could lead to short-circuiting of nerve impulses between two nerve fibres or affect the pattern of afferent nerve impulses in such a way as to synchronize the neuronal firing of their central pathways.

Operations have been devised to decompress the Gasserian ganglion or sensory root with temporary relief or to compress these structures with more lasting relief, but alcohol injection or section of the sensory root have remained the standard surgical procedures. These are now required less frequently since carbamazepine (Tegretol) 200–400 mg three times a day suppresses the pain in about 70 per cent of patients. Phenytoin (Dilantin) 100–200 mg three times a day is rather less successful. The rationale for the use of these anticonvulsant drugs is that trigeminal neuralgia may be regarded as a 'peripheral epilepsy' caused by synchronous and often repetitive discharge of the sensory neurones of the trigeminal nerve, or their central connections. Carbamazepine may rarely cause leucopenia and cases of aplastic anaemia have been reported. For this reason, patients should be warned to report for a blood count should they develop any infection. The blood may be checked every 3 months as a routine but it is doubtful whether regular blood counts really fulfil any useful function since leucopenia may appear quite suddenly. Carbamazepine may be used to tide the patient over a bout of trigeminal neuralgia and then withdrawn during a period of remission.

Glossopharyngeal Neuralgia

Glossopharyngeal neuralgia is about 100 times less common than trigeminal neuralgia and causes a similar type of lancinating pain in the ear, base of the tongue, tonsillar fossa, or beneath the angle of the jaw. The distribution is not only in the sensory area of the glossopharyngeal nerve but also of the auricular and pharyngeal branches of the vagus nerve.[40] It is provoked by swallowing, talking or coughing. If the pain does not respond to carbamazepine, intracranial section of the glossopharyngeal nerve and upper two rootlets of the vagus nerve has been recommended.

Post-herpetic Neuralgia

Herpes zoster commonly attacks the first division of the trigeminal nerve and leaves in its wake an unpleasant burning pain in the partially anaesthetic area. The pain may cause diagnostic difficulty by appearing before the rash or, on rare occasions, without any rash at all. The rash may also appear in the external auditory meatus, on the soft palate, or in the distribution of the upper cervical nerve roots. Paralysis of the third, fourth or sixth cranial nerves, or a facial palsy, may accompany the herpetic eruption (*Figure 7.3*). Post-herpetic neuralgia probably depends upon a patchy degeneration of nerve fibres which alters the pattern of nerve impulses transmitted to the nervous system so that they are misinterpreted as pain. Local measures such as the use of vibrators applied to the affected area and section of the supra-orbital and frontal nerves are rarely successful, and carbamazepine is of little help in this condition. The author's experience accords with that of Woodforde and colleagues[215] who found that the majority of patients with post-herpetic neuralgia were depressed and that antidepressant drugs, particularly amitriptyline in doses of 75–150 mg daily are helpful in relieving the pain. The intravenous infusion of 500 ml procaine 0·1–0·2 per cent has been advocated. More recently, the use of steroids in the acute phase of herpes zoster has been reported as preventing post-herpetic neuralgia without producing spread of the infection, and the local application of 40 per cent idoxuridine in dimethyl sulphoxide has been found to reduce the painful period to less than 9 days.

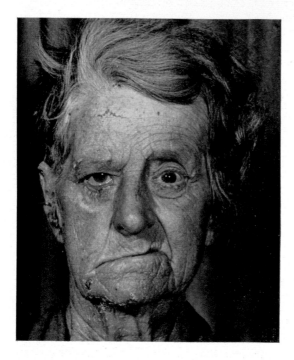

Figure 7.3. Herpes zoster affecting the external ear and upper neck with a right facial paralysis

LOCAL CRANIAL DISORDERS

Occasionally a scalp infection may give rise to pain which is described as headache. Any expanding lesion of bone which stretches the periosteum may also cause local pain. Paget's disease may be accompanied by a constant headache of the tension-vascular pattern, but a causal relationship is not certain.

REFERRED PAIN

Eyes

Imbalance of the extra-ocular muscles (heterophoria), especially convergence weakness, or refractive errors, particularly uncorrected presbyopia, may set up 'eyestrain' headache, which is a form of tension headache following visual effort. Angle-closure glaucoma may cause pain to be felt deeply in the eye and to radiate over the forehead in the distribution of the first division of the trigeminal nerve. There may not be mistiness of vision, coloured haloes seen around lights or circumcorneal injection to draw attention to the eye. Radiation of pain from eye to forehead should arouse suspicion of glaucoma in the middle-aged or elderly patient and lead to a full ophthalmological examination including measurement of the intra-ocular tension.

Pain in or behind the eye is a common feature of retrobulbar neuritis and may precede impairment of vision by a few hours or even days. The pain radiates to the frontal region of the same side. Sight becomes blurred and may be lost completely in the affected eye. The most common visual field defect is a central scotoma since the central part of the optic nerve containing fibres from the macula is most often affected by the demyelinating process. It is probable that retrobulbar neuritis is always caused by primary demyelination of the optic nerve, and more than half the patients who suffer an attack subsequently develop signs of demyelination elsewhere in the nervous system. The exact percentage of patients who progress to typical multiple sclerosis varies greatly from series to series depending upon the criteria of diagnosis and the length of follow-up.

During the acute attack, the eyeball is often tender to pressure and aches on eye movement. The optic fundi are usually normal on ophthalmoscopic examination unless the area of demyelination underlies the nerve head, when swelling of the optic disc is observed. This inflammatory oedema, termed papillitis, is said to give a reddish appearance to the disc as well as the characteristic appearance of papilloedema. Distinction between the two conditions does not present any difficulty because vision is seriously impaired or lost in papillitis, whereas there is usually no more than slight blurring of vision on head movement with papilloedema, even when the disc is grossly swollen.

Both pain and visual disturbance of retrobulbar neuritis usually respond rapidly to the use of adrenocorticotrophic hormone (ACTH). A recent controlled trial of ACTH 40 units daily given for 30 days demonstrated that all 25 patients given the active substance were relieved of pain within 48 hours, some within a few hours.[152] The control group of 25 patients continued to have pain for up to 2 weeks. Vision improved more rapidly in the treated group. At the end of 30 days, only 2 patients in the treated group were unable to read small print, compared with 12 of the untreated patients. There is evidence that demyelination responds better to ACTH than to adrenal corticosteroids, and it is possible that some substance other than cortisol, released from the adrenal cortex by ACTH, is responsible for the beneficial results. One patient of mine provided convincing evidence of the efficacy of ACTH in that pain diminished and vision returned within 24 hours of starting treatment with ACTH on three occasions. The first course of injections was ceased after about 1 week because the condition appeared to have subsided but pain and blindness returned 1 day afterwards. A second course of 2 weeks was equally effective but recurrence followed as soon as treatment was stopped. The third course was continued for 6 weeks, after which the patient remained symptom-free.

Ears, Nose and Throat

Vasomotor rhinitis is said to give rise to a mid-frontal headache. The author is rather sceptical of this statement since vasomotor rhinitis is a common disorder in Australia and affects many of his patients and colleagues (and himself) without causing headache. It does, of course, predispose to sinusitis, which causes headache in the stage of active inflammation or when the ostium of a particular sinus is obstructed.

The diagnosis of sinusitis rarely presents any difficulty when the pain and tenderness are localized to the affected frontal or maxillary sinus or sinuses and percussion over the area increases the pain. Inflammation of the ethmoid or sphenoidal sinuses gives rise to a boring pain felt deeply in the midline behind the nose. The pain of sinusitis is made worse by bending the head forwards. If the ostium to the infected sinus is patent, blowing the nose or sneezing usually evokes a throb of pain.

One or both nostrils are usually blocked and the maintenance of a clear airway by decongestants will lead to discharge of mucopurulent material from the sinuses with subsequent relief of pain in most instances. The use of vasoconstrictor nose drops or nasal spray, such as neosynephrine 0·25 per cent every 2–3 hours, instilled first with the head postured backwards over the end of a bed, and then, after some minutes, with the head upright, will clear the airway in most patients. When the airway is clear, steam inhalation, followed by the application of radiant heat to the affected area, helps to clear the ostia. If symptoms of systemic disturbance appear, antibiotics may be required but the first requirement is to ensure that sinuses are draining freely. If this cannot be accomplished by the simple measures outlined, the advice of an ear, nose and throat surgeon should be obtained. Sinusitis is often taken lightly but may be treacherous if it persists, and lead to collections of pus in the extra-dural or subdural spaces, to cerebral abscess or to spread of infection through the bloodstream.

Case Report

The following reports on a patient with frontal sinusitis leading to extradural empyema, cerebral abscess and pyaemia.

A boy aged 16 years complained of right supra-orbital pain for 10 days before he was referred to the hospital because of increasing severity of headache and vomiting over the past few days. Apart from slight stiffness of the neck, no abnormality was found on admission to hospital. CSF pressure was found to be 140 mm and the fluid contained 250 cells/mm³, half of which were polymorphonuclear, and a protein content of 90 mg/100 ml. He was considered to have a viral meningitis until a left sided epileptic seizure 1 week after admission prompted a neurological consultation. On examination, the abdominal reflexes were found to be diminished on the left side and the left plantar response was less definitely flexor than the right. Radiographs demonstrated uniform opacity of the right frontal sinus and electroencephalographic findings were typical of right frontal abscess with high voltage 2 c/s waves focal at the right precentral electrode (*Figure 7.4*). After this was confirmed by carotid arteriography, an extradural collection of pus was evacuated, followed by an operation on the frontal sinus, aspiration of an abscess in the right frontal lobe and finally aspiration of a purulent arthritis of a knee joint. The radiographic appearance of the right frontal sinus with the abscess cavity behind it is illustrated in *Figure 7.5*. The lad eventually made a complete recovery. The offending organism was staphylococcus aureus.

A mucocele may develop in one frontal sinus if the ostium of the sinus is obstructed and can slowly expand, eroding bone until it projects into the orbit, causing proptosis.

Carcinoma of the nasopharynx may invade the base of the skull, causing pain by involvement of the fifth, ninth and tenth cranial nerves.

Hippocrates warned that an association of headache with acute pain in the ear is to be dreaded 'for there is danger that the man may become delirious and die'.[4] Otitis media was mentioned in the last chapter in relation to thrombosis of the lateral sinus and 'otitic hydrocephalus'. Intracranial abscesses from middle ear disease are uncommon nowadays, but may be found in the temporal lobe or cerebellum and present with signs of raised intracranial pressure, focal neurological disturbance or meningeal irritation.

65

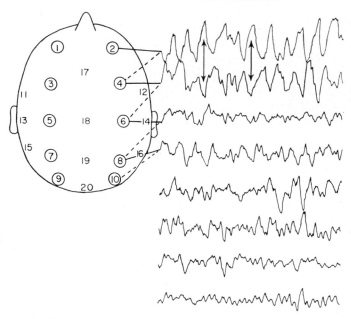

Figure 7.4. Electroencephalogram in cerebral abscess. The sketch on the left represents the head seen from above with the standard electrode placements and the origin of the tracings from the right hemisphere are indicated. High voltage slow waves are seen to arise in the right frontal region, with phase reversal (shown by arrows) demonstrating their origin from the right precentral electrode

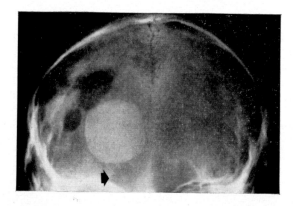

Figure 7.5. Intra-cerebral abscess arising from right frontal sinusitis (same patient as Figure 7.4). The right frontal sinus (arrowed) is less radiolucent than the left. The abscess cavity is demonstrated by the injection of radio-opaque material after drainage through the burr holes which may be seen above and lateral to it. (Case history in text)

66

Teeth

Dental caries or apical root infection can cause a neuralgic pain in the second or third divisions of the trigeminal nerve, with a constant aching component and superadded jabbing pains. The pain is made worse by hot or cold fluids in the mouth. Pains in the lower jaw are almost always of dental origin and warrant careful radiographs of the teeth as apical root infections may be missed in a routine examination. Pains in the upper jaw are commonly of dental origin but can readily be produced by maxillary sinusitis.

A common way for dental disturbance to refer pain to the upper part of the head is through dysfunction of one temporomandibular joint. If the bite is unbalanced by premature contact of one or more teeth or by loss of molar teeth on one side, or if the bite is fixed so that the normal lateral or shearing movement of mastication is impossible, the patient adopts the most convenient chewing position, which commonly throws an abnormal strain on one temporomandibular joint. This may lead to pain which is felt in front of or behind the ear on the appropriate side with radiation to the temple, over the face, and down the neck on that side, often associated with a blocked sensation in that ear (Costen's syndrome).[43] The condition is made worse by the patient becoming a chronic 'jaw clencher' if he was not one already, so that tension symptoms are set up in the temporal and other scalp muscles. Ill-fitting dentures or any other source of discomfort in biting or chewing may evoke the same symptoms. In long-standing cases crepitus may be heard or felt over the affected temporomandibular joint.

The management depends upon careful adjustment of the bite by a dental surgeon, but advice to the patient concerning relaxation of the temporal and masseter muscles is also helpful. The problem is discussed further under the heading of Tension Headache.

Neck

Degeneration of the upper cervical disc spaces or deformity of the first two or three cervical vertebrae can cause compression of the appropriate posterior roots which refer pain to the occipital region. Pain is also experienced in the neck and, if the lower cervical spine is also affected, the shoulder girdle as well. The first and second vertebrae are commonly involved in advanced rheumatoid arthritis with angulation of the odontoid process and subluxation of the joints (*Figure 7.6*). In addition to pain in the head and neck, spinal cord compression may be an indication for operative fixation of the upper cervical spine.

The contribution of changes in the lower cervical spine to generalized headache is more controversial. Kerr[102] has shown that stimulation of the upper cervical nerve roots may refer pain to the trigeminal distribution, but there is no known means of referral of pain to the head from the lower cervical spine. One sees many patients with cervical spondylosis complaining of pain in the neck and shoulders,

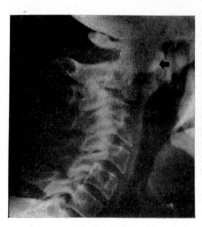 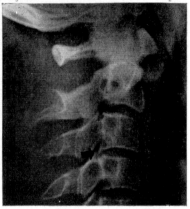

Figure 7.6. Deformity of the upper cervical spine in rheumatoid arthritis. The odontoid process (arrowed) is angulated forwards. The patient presented with occipital headache and signs of spinal cord compression

Figure 7.7. Mild degenerative changes in the cervical spine associated with headache referred to the eye. Disc spaces between the third and fourth, and fifth and sixth cervical vertebrae are slightly narrowed with posterior projection of osteophytes at the upper level (arrowed). (Case history in text)

with paraesthesiae in the hands, who do not have headache. When headache is a symptom of such patients, its quality and associations are usually those of muscle-contraction (tension) headache, which may be initiated by concern over their neck condition or may be independent of it. It has been postulated that cervical spondylosis may damage the periarterial nerve plexus of the vertebral artery by osteophytes impinging on it, and hence set up diffuse headache, but this concept remains unproven. The occasional dramatic relief of headache by cervical manipulation must be balanced against those patients whose headache is unimproved and whose neck pain may be made worse by manipulative procedures. There are a few whose radiological signs of spondylosis are limited to the lower cervical spine but whose headache appears to be brought on or aggravated by neck movement and who are relieved by cervical traction.

Case Report

The following presents a case of cervical spondylosis with referral of pain to the head and face.

A medical colleague aged 42 years had been subject to recurrent attacks of pain in the right shoulder since he was a student. After some years pain was experienced in the neck as well as the shoulder during these attacks and he noticed crepitus in the neck. At the age of 33 years he developed right sciatic pain with numbness of the sole, and a degenerated lumbosacral disc was removed by laminectomy. His neck and shoulder pain continued to recur several times a year. At the age of 41 years he noticed pain above, behind and below the right eye after playing golf. He attributed this to twisting his neck in fixing the golf ball with his left eye. The pain then became daily and was referred from the eye to the temple and ear on the right side. The pain was made worse by neck movement or by the vibration and jolting of car or air travel. When the pain became severe he had to hold his neck to the left, so as to extend the right side of the neck, to obtain relief. No abnormality was found on examination apart from stiffness and crepitus in the neck. Electroencephalography was within normal limits. Radiographs of the skull and sinuses were normal but those of the cervical spine disclosed degenerative changes at the disc space between the third and fourth cervical vertebrae (*Figure 7.7*). A right carotid arteriogram was done in view of the distribution of the pain and was normal. The headache eased gradually during a course of cervical traction. It has not recurred in the past year although he has had further episodes of neck pain.

PSYCHOGENIC HEADACHE

The importance of psychological factors in migraine and tension headache is mentioned in the appropriate chapters. The term 'psychogenic headache' is used to describe the association of headache with florid psychiatric disturbance such as acute depression, schizophrenia or hysteria. Headache may be incorporated into the delusional system of such patients. There is no way in which any mechanism can be postulated for such headaches incorporating peripheral pain pathways. The headache is a concept of disordered thought processes and appears or disappears with the mental state which engendered it.

Case Report

The following presents a case of headache in paranoid schizophrenia.

A man aged 43 years had suffered from constant bilateral headache, '7 days a week and 24 hours a day' for the past 7 years. He had been a champion boxer in earlier days and considered that his frontal lobes had been damaged by boxing injuries. He stated that he had been 'bashed up by the underworld' thousands of times and that his recent head injuries had brought back memories of head injuries 20 years ago. He said that the underworld, under the leadership of a prominent judge, had been squirting cyanide through water pistols into his bedroom and placing rubber masks over his head. He felt 'boiled up' and 'filled with hate' and had the sensation of an ulcer in his head. His present headache was attributed to cyanide administered per rectum while he was unconscious from a pellet-gun wound.

ATYPICAL FACIAL PAIN

Depressed or anxious patients may present with a constant aching pain in the face which defies analysis, and does not respond to conventional headache remedies, or even to blockade or section of what would appear to be the appropriate cranial nerves. It could be said that it bears the same relationship to 'lower half headache' as tension headache does to migraine. The pain is commonly unilateral and is felt deeply in the angle of the nose or in the cheek. It is constant and boring in quality and may spread diffusely to other areas of the head or neck at times of exacerbation. There is often a history of some minor dental procedure or a blow to the face from which the onset of the pain is dated. The mechanism remains obscure but the present approach is to regard atypical facial pain as a depressive symptom[205], and treatment with amitriptyline, imipramine or mono-amine oxidase inhibitors provides complete or partial relief in most patients. Electroconvulsive therapy has been used with success in resistant patients.

Case Report

The following presents an atypical facial pain.

A man aged 43 years had suffered a single major epileptic seizure 10 years previously. Shortly after this the left upper gum started to ache and he was treated by washing out the left maxillary sinus and removing the nasal septum. Pain has persisted since then, starting in the left upper gum near the midline and radiating upwards to the left nostril and the left cheek under the eye. It was barely noticeable in the early morning and became progressively worse during the day. A left carotid arteriogram and CSF examination in another hospital were found to be normal. A radical antrostomy did not provide relief. The left infra-orbital nerve was blocked with alcohol, and finally sectioned, without any benefit. The left cheek, nostril and upper lip have felt numb since then but pain has remained in the anaesthetic areas.

He had been subject to typical right-sided migraine headaches which had recurred every three months throughout his life. He said that he was a tense, worrying man who had felt depressed ever since his fit

10 years ago. He was treated with amitriptyline 25 mg three times daily and after 2 weeks said that the pain was reduced in severity and that he felt much brighter and could face life again. After four months' treatment, the pain was still present but he felt that he could now live with it satisfactorily. He had found that deliberately relaxing his jaw eliminated his facial pain.

Over a period of 5 years his pain gradually returned to its former intensity. It was not benefited by intracranial section of the second and third divisions of the trigeminal nerve, by increasing the dose of amitriptyline to 150 mg daily or by monoamine oxidase inhibitors. The sphenopalatine ganglion was blocked with cocaine and the stellate ganglion was injected with xylocaine, producing a Horner's syndrome, without any change in the facial pain. Dr. T. Torda infiltrated the upper cervical posterior roots, resulting in analgesia from the limits of the trigeminal distribution down to the fourth cervical segment without improvement. On another occasion Dr. Torda induced an epidural block of posterior roots which extended from the fourth cervical segment down to the second thoracic segment but the pain persisted at the height of analgesia. Electroconvulsive therapy administered to the right hemisphere on 8 occasions over a period of 3 weeks did not help. A modified leucotomy is now being considered.

POST-TRAUMATIC HEADACHE

The incidence of post-traumatic headache varies in different series from 33 to 80 per cent.[29] The problem which exercises the neurologist is to assign the correct proportion of organic and psychological factors in each particular instance. Brenner, Friedman, Merritt and Denny-Brown[29] found that post-traumatic headache lasting more than 2 months was uncommon in those patients who were only dazed and were not disorientated after the injury, and those without post-traumatic amnesia. It was significantly higher in those with laceration of the scalp and in those of a nervous disposition before the accident, with symptoms of anxiety after the accident or with occupational difficulties or pending litigation. There was no correlation with the duration of coma, disorientation or post-traumatic amnesia when these were present, or with EEG abnormalities during the first week, skull fracture or the finding of blood in the CSF. These authors quote earlier work by Friedman and Brenner which showed that patients with localized post-traumatic headache were very sensitive to intravenous histamine which reproduced the characteristic headache. These findings suggest that some post-traumatic headache is of intracranial origin (worsened by histamine) some is of extracranial origin (following laceration of the scalp) and some is of psychosomatic origin (worsened by anxiety and

71

concern about litigation). The settlement of the legal aspects of the matter does not always lead to disappearance of symptoms and return to work. Balla and Moraitis[14] followed up 82 patients, 41 of whom suffered from headache, after industrial or traffic accidents. They found that 21 patients had not returned to work 2 years after financial settlement. Those who did return to work usually did so within a year.

Ellard[64] has summarized the psychological reactions he has encountered in patients with a compensable injury as follows:

Attitudinal pathosis

A patient who does not seek to be healed but to be justified. He is not incapacitated by symptoms but has a grievance and believes that he cannot work because he has been dealt with unjustly.

Schizophrenic reaction

This is commonly paranoid with feelings of persecution by doctors, solicitors and even the law courts. Less commonly, a neurotic illness develops extraordinary features, such as the man who had a bump on the head and thereafter wore glasses with one red lens and one green lens and could walk only with the aid of a stick adorned by a wheel at one end and a bicycle bell at the other. Ellard comments that patients who habitually wear pyjama trousers under their ordinary trousers seem to pursue a particularly malignant course.

Bizarre hypochondriasis

A group of patients who before injury were fitness fanatics, narcissistic and preoccupied with health foods and sporting activities. They commonly describe their headache in an exaggerated manner and are often diagnosed as hysterical.

Traumatic neurosis

Here the accident may have symbolic significance, perhaps of a sexual nature, but more commonly the patient's anxiety is conditioned by the accident, like the woman who could only tolerate being driven in a car if she huddled under a rug in the rear compartment drinking brandy. Such patients may respond to behaviour therapy.

Depression

Many patients who become depressed are of compulsive personality in whom work has become an important defence mechanism. Typical depressive symptoms follow deprivation of their normal working pattern.

Compensation neurosis

Depressive symptoms are usually overshadowed by those of anxiety. The patient often becomes aggressive at work as well as at home. Hysterical manifestations may become superimposed. The total amount of disability is usually greater than the sum of its parts.

Malingering

The paradox of the man who remains sick because of the hope of financial reward.

Ellard stresses the need to assess each patient in the light of his racial, cultural and educational background as well as his premorbid personality. The patient with an excessive psychological reaction to injury looks well in spite of his description of suffering. There is a lack of motivation to get well and his attitude to treatment is unusual and may be resentful.

In the present state of knowledge, headache following injury cannot be classified with certainty in any one group. It is probable that there are four distinct types of post-traumatic headache, with overlap between the groups.

(1) Intracranial Vascular Headache

It is generally accepted that concussion is followed by dilatation of intracranial vessels, giving rise to a pulsating headache which is made worse by head movement, jolting, coughing, sneezing and straining. This type of headache may persist for months after head injury, without any obvious neurological signs being present. It may be associated with other symptoms of organic origin, such as giddiness on looking upwards or on lying down with the head to one side or the other (benign positional vertigo). The same type of headache may develop, or intensify, in the case of subdural haematoma arising as a result of head injury.

(2) Extracranial Vascular Headache

It is not uncommon for patients who have experienced local damage to the scalp overlying a main extracranial vessel to become subject to periodic headache in the distribution of that vessel. Such headaches have been called post-traumatic migraine, since they recur with the periodicity of migraine and may be associated with nausea and photophobia. Jabbing pains may also rise from any scalp nerve damaged by the blow, or subsequent development of scar tissue. Ligation and section of the affected nerve and vessel may

73

be helpful in abolishing this syndrome. Apart from surgical measures, the management is the same as for migraine.

(3) Pain in the Neck and Occipital Region from Injury to the Upper Cervical Spine

The part played by 'whiplash injury' of the cervical spine is difficult to assess in the absence of definite radiological changes. Some patients respond to the local application of heat and cervical traction or the local injection of procaine and hydrocortisone into tender areas of the musculature of the neck. The majority show features of anxiety and their symptoms resemble those of muscle-contraction headache.

(4) Muscle-contraction ('Tension') Headache

It has been amply pointed out in the medical literature that multiple symptoms may follow minor head injuries where compensation or litigation is involved and that self-employed or professional men return to work more rapidly than employees after head injury, and that sporting injuries are not usually followed by disability. Any tendency to anxiety or depression appears to be accentuated by head injury, and the personality of the patient before the accident plays a large part in the way that he reacts to injury. Some post-traumatic headaches have all the qualities of tension headache and respond, at least in part, to the use of tranquillizing and antidepressant drugs. The tendency to this form of headache is often engendered by that natural worry which attaches to the possibility of brain damage and is reinforced by some legal advisors who instruct their clients not to resume work or normal activities until the case is settled. The concept of accident neurosis has been discussed in detail in two lectures by Miller.[136]

The great difficulty in handling patients with post-traumatic headache is to differentiate the organic from the psychogenic components. It seems undeniable that some post-traumatic headache is of organic origin, in the sense that the control of cranial vessels has become more unstable, and cranial arteries have become more susceptible to painful dilatation since injury.[192] It requires an unbiased approach on the part of the physician and a careful assessment of each patient's personality and his headache pattern to ensure that justice is done to his legal claim and that treatment is appropriate to his variety of headache.

74

8—Muscle-Contraction ('Tension')
Headache

In peace there's nothing so becomes a man
As modest stillness and humility:
But when the blast of war blows in our ears,
Then imitate the action of the tiger;
Stiffen the sinews, summon up the blood,
Disguise fair nature with hard-favour'd rage;
Then lend the eye a terrible aspect;
. . . . let the brow o'erwhelm it . . . .
Now set the teeth and stretch the nostril wide . . . .

King Henry V, III. i

The staring eyes, furrowed brows and clenched teeth are appropriate enough in a man preparing for battle. A grimly set visage can be quite a handicap when it is the constant accompaniment of everyday life. When the sinews are stiffened in reaction to a crisis, physiological mechanisms 'summon up the blood' to supply the contracting muscles. When the muscles of a tense patient cannot stop contracting, the flow of blood through them may not be sufficient to prevent pain and herein may lie the cause of tension headache.

CLINICAL FEATURES

Incidence, Age and Sex Distribution

Most people have probably been aware of a dull headache at some time of their lives after exposure to glare, flickering light, eyestrain, noise or a succession of harassing incidents. The number of persons who often experience such headaches must be considerable, judging from the sale of headache tablets and powders. The incidence of tension headaches which are frequent enough to warrant referral to a neurological clinic is almost as great as that of migraine. Over a period of 2½ years, 1,152 patients were referred to one out-patient clinic with the complaint of headache. Of these 612 suffered from migraine and 466 from tension headache.[121]

75

It is well known that migraine often begins in childhood but it is surprising to find that about 15 per cent of patients with tension headache also remember that their symptoms started before the age of 10 years (*Figure 8.1*). The condition may be intractable and persist throughout life. Many patients have suffered from headaches almost every day for 10, 20 or 30 years (*Figure 8.2*). As in the case of migraine, roughly 75 per cent of patients with chronic tension headache are women.

Family History

Some 18 per cent of patients with tension headache give a family history of migraine,[113] which is much the same as for the general population. However, a family background of some form of headache is found in the history of 40 per cent of tension headache patients.[76]

Past Health

There is no evidence that allergic disorders, childhood vomiting attacks or other disabilities are more common in patients complaining of tension headache than in the general community.

Site of Headache

Muscle-contraction headache is bilateral in about 90 per cent of patients.[76] It may be unilateral in patients who have imbalance of the bite. If a patient has a few back teeth missing on one side, or if the teeth cannot move freely from side to side, the bite is locked or distorted. The patient tends to chew on one side, throwing the strain onto one or other temporomandibular joint, so that the pain is felt in front of the ear and radiates over the temple.

Chronic jaw-clenchers commonly complain of pain over the contracting temporal and masseter muscles. The constant frowners have bifrontal headache and the 'stiff-necks' describe occipital pain. These sites may flow into one another so that the patient feels pain 'all over the head'.

Quality of Headache

The pain is usually dull and persistent in tension headache, and undulates in intensity during the day. It is often described as a feeling of heaviness, pressure or tightness rather than pain and may extend like a band around the head. Some patients experience sudden jabs of pain on one side or at the back of the head superimposed on a general background of discomfort. About one-quarter

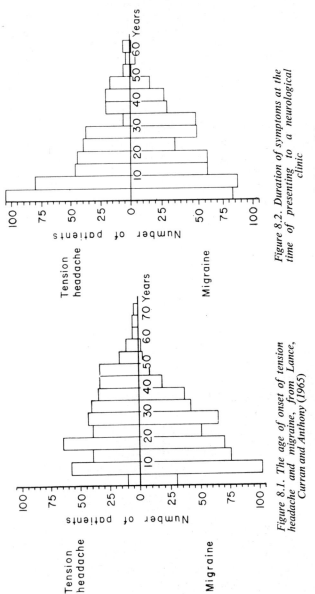

Figure 8.1. The age of onset of tension headache and migraine, from Lance, Curran and Anthony (1965)

Figure 8.2. Duration of symptoms at the time of presenting to a neurological clinic

(Reproduced by courtesy of the Editor of the Medical Journal of Australia)

of tension-headache patients, whose headaches become severe and assume a pulsating quality at times, form a group intermediate between muscle-contraction headache and migraine which is called 'tension-vascular headache'.[120] It is not uncommon for the headache to be throbbing on awakening but to settle down to its usual uniform character on starting the day's activities. About 10 per cent of patients with tension headache are also subject to frank migraine.

Time and Mode of Onset

In milder cases, the headache develops during or after recognizable stress. It may thus arise as a housewife gets her children off to school and her husband off to work; or while a driver battles with peak-hour traffic; or when the business executive is trying to juggle interviews and telephone conversations with the knowledge that he has not read the agenda for that meeting at 5 p.m. In more severe cases, the headache comes on in anticipation of some unpleasant situation, such as a distasteful interview. Contemplation of the day's tasks may be enough to start a headache while travelling to work by train. Immediately before the projected battle with Tweedledee, Tweedledum remarked 'I'm very brave generally, only today I happen to have a headache'.

In the most chronic form, the patient either awakens with the headache or notices it shortly after getting up and it remains throughout the day, without regard to the emotional content of the day's activities. Some 10 per cent of patients, not necessarily those who are depressed, may be woken up by tension-vascular headache between 1 a.m. and 4 a.m. in the manner of a migrainous patient.

Frequency and Duration

Of 466 patients attending our neurological clinic for the treatment of tension headache, the headache recurred less than ten times each month in 48 patients, from 10 to 30 times each month in 64 patients and was present every day in the remaining 354 patients.[120] Friedman and his colleagues[76] found that 50 per cent of their patients experienced headaches every day. It is apparent that those patients attending clinics are those who are most severely affected and that figures from clinics do not necessarily reflect the pattern of tension headache as seen by the general practitioner. The spectrum of tension headache extends from headaches of 1 hour's duration recurring every few months to a perpetual unremitting ache present 'all day and every day'.

Associated Phenomena

Muscle-contraction headache is not accompanied by any of the focal neurological symptoms which add a distinctive character to most attacks of migraine. There is often a constant mild photophobia, not severe enough to make the patient retreat to a darkened room but often sufficient to encourage the wearing of sunglasses on all but the gloomiest day. Other symptoms are those of an anxiety state. Slight nausea may be present in the early mornings, or when the headache is severe, but vomiting is rare. Giddiness or light headedness usually indicates a tendency to over-breathe in times of anxiety. The patient often speaks of difficulty in concentrating and a lack of interest in work or hobbies. There may be more flagrant depressive symptoms which are attributed to the presence of headache. Pain under the left breast, pain in the back or coccygeal region, and indigestion are other psychosomatic symptoms commonly associated with tension headache. The patient may awaken with a bruised sensation inside the mouth lateral to the posterior upper molar tooth as the result of extreme mandibular movements during sleep.[66]

Underlying, Precipitating, Aggravating and Relieving Factors

It is deceptively easy to think of patients with tension headache as having an inadequate personality. This is certainly true of some patients who are ill-equipped by nature or education to cope with life's ramifications, but there are others who have considerable achievements to their credit. It may be that the meticulous energetic personality which has made a man prey to tension headache has also made him a leader in industry. A recent review by Martin, Rome and Swanson[132] concludes: 'There does not seem to be a single psychologic determinant productive of muscle-contraction headaches. Multiple conflicts are usually evident in patients . . . poorly repressed hostility is often evident, but unresolved dependency needs and psychosexual conflicts are also frequently present. . . . However, it seems that the psychophysiologic expression at somatization of anxiety in the form of increased skeletal-muscle tension is uniformly present in cases of muscle-contraction headache.'

In the author's own experience, approximately one-third of patients with tension headache have symptoms of depression.[120] Most are conscious of the fact that they are never really relaxed and are rarely elated. Many patients with tension headache are 'born two drinks down on life'.

79

There may be obvious trigger factors for tension headache but in many patients the headache is not limited to times of emotional overload. The headache is usually made worse by any superadded anxiety, stress, noise or glare. It is aggravated by the administration of vasocontrictor agents and improved by vasodilators.[28,145] A headache which is relieved by the taking of alcohol is almost invariably of the tension variety, whereas most vascular headaches become more severe. Muscle-contraction headache is usually relieved by aspirin or preparations which combine caffeine with analgesics, but recurs after some hours. This may lead to repeated self-medication with subsequent risk of habituation and toxicity.

Physical Examination

Formal neurological examination is usually normal, but signs of muscular over-contraction are found in the majority of patients. Some patients look the part, with deep wrinkles on face and forehead where time has etched their personality traits. The temporal and masseter muscles may stand out and twitch, and the hands may clench the chair firmly or the fingers move restlessly during the inverview. Other patients may have a bland appearance which is impassive due to muscular rigidity and rarely softens into a smile.

A simple test of the ability to relax is to lift the patient's arm up in one's hands and to tell the patient that he or she must imagine it is resting on an armchair (*Figure 8.3*). The aim is to let the limb go completely loose so that when the examiner's hands are removed the arm will flop lifelessly downwards to the patient's side. In fact, the vast majority of tension-headache patients assure the examiner that the arm is completely relaxed and are surprised to find that it still rests on the imaginary armchair once the supporting hands are taken away (*Figure 8.4*). Similar to the 'armchair sign' is the 'invisible pillow'. A patient who is instructed to let the head loll back in the examiner's hands will frequently maintain the head rigidly in position above the couch (*Figure 8.5*) and can only put it down by a conscious voluntary extension movement of the neck. It should be possible to relax the legs so that they can be bent freely at the knees or rolled from side to side. Most patients with tension headache are quite unable to do this. It should be possible to let the jaw hang down so that it can be moved rapidly up and down through a small range by the examiner. Most tension headache patients hold the jaw so rigidly that the whole head moves with the mandible (*Figure 8.6*). Auscultation over the temporal muscles will confirm the presence of inappropriate contraction.

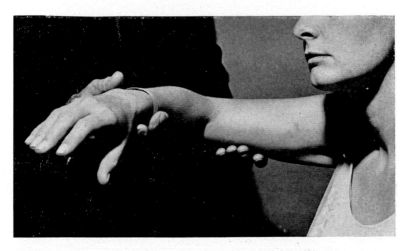

Figure 8.3. Testing the ability of a patient with tension headache to relax skeletal muscles at will. The patient is instructed to let the arm go loose in the examiner's hand as though it were resting on an armchair

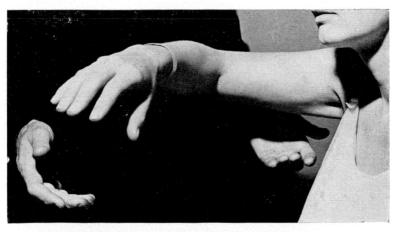

Figure 8.4. When the examiner's hand is removed, the patient's arm remains on the invisible armchair. The patient had been unaware that the arm was not completely relaxed

G

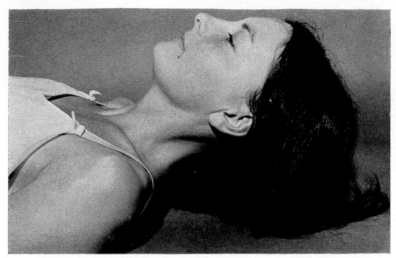

Figure 8.5. Difficulty in relaxing the neck muscles in a patient with tension headache The examiner's hands have just been removed from a position where they were 'supporting' the patient's head. The neck muscles continued to contract so that the head remained elevated after the hands were withdrawn

Figure 8.6. The ability to relax the jaw muscles can be tested by attempting to move the jaw rapidly up and down without displacing the head. In most patients with tension headache, the head moves with the jaw which is held rigidly

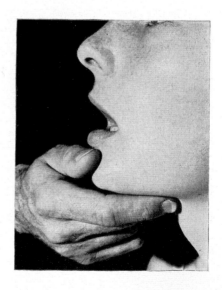

82

The constant driving from above of spinal mechanisms may induce such hyperactivity of stretch reflexes that the examiner may feel a sensation akin to the rigidity of Parkinson's disease on manipulating a joint through its range of movement. If the patient also has an exaggerated physiological tremor as part of an anxiety state, then the similarity to Parkinson's disease may be heightened by the superimposition of a cog-wheel effect on the increased muscle tone. Indeed, the mechanism is probably a functional or reversible overactivity of descending motor pathways which are thrown permanently into action in Parkinson's disease by anatomical and biochemical changes.

The elicitation of these physical signs of nervous tension is important not only for diagnosis but also to demonstrate to the patient that muscular hyperactivity is present, and to prepare the way for relaxation exercises as a part of treatment.

THE MECHANISM OF
MUSCLE-CONTRACTION HEADACHE

A constant factor in the production of tension headache appears to be the inability to relax the muscles of the face, scalp and neck, but not everyone with these characteristics develops headache. There is some additional element in the headache patient, which is not clearly understood, but which is probably hereditary. It may have to do with vascular reactivity in the muscles of scalp and neck, or with the accumulation of pain-provoking substances in muscle, or with both.

Recordings of the pulsation from scalp arteries show that vascular reactions in tension headache are the reverse of those seen in migraine. Whereas the scalp vessels dilate in migraine attacks, the amplitude of their pulsation is reduced in tension headache.[197] This suggests that patients are unable to 'summon up the blood' necessary to nourish the hyperactive scalp musculature. The small vessels of the conjunctiva have been examined and photographed during tension headache and have been seen to constrict as long as a frontal headache lasts.[145] This unseemly vasoconstriction may be partly responsible for tension headache, since the pain becomes worse with vasoconstrictor agents such as noradrenaline and ergotamine, and is relieved temporarily by the inhalation of amyl nitrite or the administration of various vasodilator drugs, including alcohol.[28,145] To test the vasoconstrictive hypothesis, a research group in New York injected a radioactive sodium preparation into the muscles at the back of the neck and checked its rate of clearance during severe occipital headache.[142] Surprisingly, they found that clearance was greater than it was in headache-free periods. At first sight this appears to be evidence against constriction of muscular arteries, but this interpretation need not be correct, because the studies were made in patients with headache of fluctuating intensity when headache was severe, thus resembling the description of 'tension-vascular headache' rather than the milder pressure sensations of the usual muscle-contraction headache.

The possibility of changes in plasma levels of serotonin, noradrenaline or other humoral agents in tension headache has not been investigated, as far as the author is aware, and it is possible that chemical changes may take place either systemically, or locally in muscles or their vessels, which sensitize end-organs to pain perception. Most tension headaches respond readily, if temporarily, to aspirin. The intraperitoneal injection of aspirin in man will prevent the pain which is induced by the intraperitoneal injection of bradykinin, whereas the same dose given intravenously is ineffective.[126] This suggests that aspirin analgesia in man may be due to blockade of pain receptors at the periphery, and that pains which are responsive to aspirin may depend upon some chemical mediator such as bradykinin. It is also possible that the interpretation of sensory patterns may be different in the patient with muscle-contraction headache. Many patients are introspective and have a low pain threshold in that they may complain of other uncomfortable sensations in different parts of the body. The cause of pain, of the constriction of scalp arteries and conjunctival arterioles in tension headache, and of increased blood-flow in some patients with tension or tension-vascular headache still has to be elucidated, quite apart from the complex psychological tangle which may underlie the observable manifestations in the head and neck.

TREATMENT OF TENSION HEADACHE

Most accounts of the treatment of tension headache correctly emphasize the psychological management of the patient. This is a sound general principle but it is rarely sufficient to cure a patient of headache. The problems of many patients are either inapparent or insoluble. Many patients say that they have not got a care in the world apart from their headache, whereas others have persistent symptoms of anxiety or depression. It is often possible to make simple suggestions about the day's routine which may ease mental strain considerably. Minor adjustments may improve efficiency and make life easier, but there are some problems which no amount of discussion will solve. There are advocates of formal psychotherapy in the treatment of tension headache but the time required makes this impractical for most patients. Hypnotism may be useful in a suggestible patient but it is an art practised by few medical practitioners.

Most patients suffering from chronic muscle-contraction headache suspect that they have a cerebral tumour or other serious intracranial disorder. The first step in treatment is to give patients a good hearing and careful examination, to give them confidence that their complaint is being taken seriously and that the doctor is not jumping to a facile

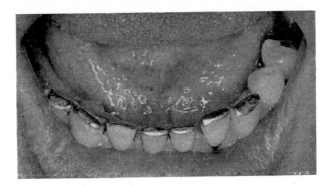

Figure 8.7. Dental restoration required by a patient because her habit of clenching her jaws had worn away the tooth enamel

conclusion in order to prescribe a tranquillizer and move on to the next patient. It is often advisable to support one's clinical opinion by arranging for an electroencephalogram and radiography of the skull and chest to provide for the patients some objective evidence that their fears are groundless.

The second step in treatment is to demonstrate that the scalp and facial muscles are indeed contracting for much of the time without reason. This can be achieved partly by questions at the end of history taking. Do your friends comment that you always look serious or worried? Do you find yourself clenching your jaws, grinding your teeth, making a tight fist with your hands? The answers to these questions can be quite surprising. Some patients have had to seek dental attention because their teeth are tender or chipped from unremitting pressure of their jaws (*Figure 8.7*). The author has had patients who have broken their dentures repeatedly by the same mechanism. Some state that they notice their fingers flexed firmly even on awakening from sleep. Every[66] has drawn attention to the nocturnal fang-sharpening movements of the jaw which occur during sleep as an indication of repressed aggression. The latter syndrome may be recognized by the association of chronic headache with pain in the temporomandibular joints and jaw muscles and a raw, tender spot on the buccal mucosa opposite the posterior part of the upper gum, which results from excessive lateral movement of the mandible during sleep. This disorder responds to psychological management rather than measures directed solely to the correction of malocclusion.

The presence of unnecessary muscular contraction can be shown to the patient at the end of physical examination. Most are unable to relax the jaw muscles so that the jaw can be moved freely by the physician. They are unable to let the head loll back when the shoulders are supported since the neck muscles remain rigid. They cannot permit their elevated arm to fall limply to the couch when requested by the examiner.

Once patients have appreciated their inability to 'switch off', the way is open to a discussion of relaxation exercises along the lines suggested by Jacobsen,[97] simplified for daily use at an appropriate time. When the house is finally quiet, after the children have left for school, the tense housewife can lie down on a comfortable bed for 5 or 10 minutes and run through a simple sequence of 'exercises'. The legs are lifted one at a time, held up for 30 seconds, then the muscles relaxed so that the leg slumps heavily on to the bed. Each arm is then raised above the bed and, after a brief period, allowed to drop lifelessly downward. The head is lifted off the pillow then permitted to flop back. The forehead is then relaxed, the eyes closed and the jaw allowed to droop open. If patients are able to accomplish complete relaxation, they should stay for some minutes with muscles flaccid in a posture determined by gravity. It will then be possible for them to acquire the technique of partial relaxation if they feel themselves becoming taut during the day. As soon as the characteristic pressure sensation appears in the forehead, temples or neck, it can be recognized, and the 'switching off' process started locally in the muscles affected, even while the day's duties are continued. If this aim is realized, the well motivated individual may require no other treatment, and remain free of headaches.

The majority find it hard to obey these simple instructions and may be helped by a physiotherapist, or a sympathetic husband or wife, in the initial stages. The application of hot packs to the site of headache, and vibrating or massaging the affected muscles, is a helpful preliminary to relaxation. Pressing the leg down hard into the bed or pulling the arm firmly against someone's hand until the subject feels fatigued may pave the way for subsequent relaxation.

86

The patient should be taught to contract each muscle group separately, to see and feel the muscle contract, then deliberately and suddenly to relax the muscle and see the muscle belly subside. The process of relaxation is an active one, to be acquired by practice, and does not come easily to most patients. Patients must be able to distinguish between the sensation of a contracting muscle and of a relaxed muscle so that they can run through each muscle group when practising on their own and ensure that complete relaxation is achieved. An observer can check that muscles are relaxed by putting a hand under the subject's knee and lifting it suddenly to ensure that the knee flexes without active resistance, or by rolling the patient's thigh to and fro to make sure that the foot flails limply with each movement. The arm can be picked up and shaken to see that it flops about 'like a rag doll'. The jaw can be moved up and down rapidly to ascertain that there is no palpable muscle resistance. These manoeuvres may sound artless but are well worthwhile as a physiological approach to the common problem of nervous tension. If patients can avoid expressing their emotions by useless overaction of muscles, they can lose their headaches even if their psychological pattern remains unchanged.

Correction of various physical factors may be necessary to help patients reach their goal of muscular relaxation. Correction of a refractive error, or orthoptic treatment for a latent ocular imbalance, may remove the factor of eye-strain which sets up a pattern of wasteful muscle activity. Dental treatment may be important to open a closed bite, restore a chewing surface, or improve dentures so that the bite is evenly distributed. Cervical traction may be useful if neck pain from degenerated intervertebral discs is triggering the tension headache.

Case Report

The following illustrates the relief of chronic tension headache by the use of relaxation exercises.

A school-teacher aged 49 years had been subject to headaches 4 or 5 days every week for 23 years. The sensation was described as a discomfort behind the forehead and eyes, which became more severe about once a month, when he felt mildly nauseated. There were no migrainous features about the headache, which came on at about midday and persisted through the afternoon, made worse by glare or concentration. He was a bachelor who had looked after his aged father until he died two years previously. He had no obvious problems but he stated he had a meticulous nature and people commented on his frowning, since he had always found it hard to relax. He was given a prescription for amitriptyline, and relaxation exercises were explained to him. He then returned to the country town where he lived and practised the exercises assiduously. The frequency of his headaches diminished to once a week or once a fortnight and he wrote to say that he had not had his prescription filled as he found that he remained virtually free of headaches as long as he continued his daily period of relaxation.

Ideally it should never be necessary to prescribe any medication in tension headache. Evaluation of any personal problem and helping the patient to overcome it, explanation of the mechanism of headache and the demonstration of muscular relaxation should be sufficient to prevent further headaches. Unfortunately, it does not work out like this, possibly because not enough is known about all the factors involved in the mechanism, and possibly because many patients are quite unable to relax even when shown how to do so.

> Bar bi turates
> Have you any pull?
> Yes sir, yes sir,
> A waiting-room full.
> One for the master,
> And one for the dame,
> And one for the doctor,
> Whose symptoms are the same.
>
> Adapted from 'Baa baa black sheep'—Anon.

In 1964, a trial was undertaken at our clinic to assess the effect of various drugs on 280 patients who were subject to tension headache for at least 10 days of each month.[120] The majority (239) of these patients experienced headaches daily. The headaches had been present for over 5 years in 211 patients and for more than 20 years in 111 patients. It was found that the use of sedatives alone (usually amylobarbitone), vasodilator drugs alone or a combination of the two, gave a response which was no different on statistical analysis from that to placebo. The muscle-relaxing drug, orphenadrine, and the migraine prophylactic drug, methysergide, were of no benefit. Improvement was obtained with the antidepressants amitriptyline (Elavil, Laroxyl, Tryptanol, Tryptizol) and imipramine (Tofranil) as well as with the tranquillizing agents chlordiazepoxide (Librium) and diazepam (Valium) and Bellergal (a proprietary product containing ergotamine tartrate 0·3 mg, phenobarbitone 20 mg and belladonna alkaloids 0·1 mg). A double-blind controlled cross-over trial was carried out with amitriptyline, which confirmed that its action did not depend upon any placebo effect. Of the patients starting the trial, 47 did not report to the clinic again after a trial of only one drug. Of the 233 who were given a number of preparations, 74 per cent improved on one or other form of medication.

As a result of this trial it has been my practice to give patients a trial period of 1 month on diazepam 5 mg three times daily if they are simply tense and anxious, or to use amitriptyline 25 mg three times daily if they are also depressed. In either instance, the patient is recommended to take one-half tablet three times daily for the first few days, since diazepam may cause drowsiness and ataxia in some people and amitriptyline may produce drowsiness, tremor, dryness of the mouth and gain in weight. It is advisable not to give amitriptyline to patients with glaucoma because of its atropine-like side-effects. Amitriptyline is not only useful in depressed patients. Of the 98 patients treated with amitriptyline in our clinical trial, 58 improved substantially, and only 18 of these had symptoms of depression. Some 7 per cent of patients are unable to tolerate amitriptyline, but it is worth a trial in any patient with chronic headache. It may be an advantage to give the full daily dosage of amitriptyline before the patient retires for the night. This may prevent drowsiness during the day, help insomnia, and does not interfere with the long-term antidepressant action. Patients who respond satisfactorily lose their headaches or notice substantial improvement from 2 to 10 days after starting treatment and it is then suggested that they continue treatment for at least 6 months and then wean off the medication slowly over a period of 2–3 months. If headaches return after treatment is stopped they usually recur after 2–14 days.

If patients do not improve after a month's trial of diazepam or amitriptyline, then the second line of defence, chlordiazepoxide for the anxious patient and imipramine for the depressed patient, or a combination of both may be tried. There are some patients whose headaches persist in spite of all measures outlined so far, and warrant referral to a psychiatrist. It may be urged that all patients with muscle-contraction headache should be referred to a psychiatrist in the first instance. This is certainly the author's policy with any patient who shows signs of serious mental disturbance, but it is not practical for every tense patient to be seen by a psychiatrist, nor would it be desirable because many patients are resentful of the implication of mental illness. The majority can be managed along the lines which have been suggested; but there are some who benefit greatly from psychiatric treatment, and the author can remember a number of his own patients who have resisted his primitive psycho-therapy, relaxation exercises and polypharmacy yet have improved after a spell of psychiatric treatment in hospital. A balanced account of the psychiatric approach to tension headache has recently been presented by Martin and Rome.[131]

9—Migraine

CLINICAL FEATURES

Incidence

Migraine is a common disorder, but just how common has been a subject of dispute in the past. One of the main difficulties in all surveys has been the definition of migraine because of the wide variation in the nature, frequency and severity of attacks. Some individuals who have only one or two attacks of migraine in their lives could hardly be included as 'sufferers from migraine'. On the other hand, there are patients who have less severe forms of headache, particularly of the tension variety, who are anxious to upgrade their symptoms and acquire the prestige of being a migraineur, who might unwittingly inflate the result of any survey. A survey of neurological disease in the English city of Carlisle found that 3·3 per cent of the community was subject to migraine and that another 3 per cent complained of other forms of chronic headache which were sufficiently frequent and severe to cause loss of time from work or school.[30] This survey was carefully carried out and it appears to be a realistic estimate.

Bille[23] studied a group of almost 9000 Swedish children and found that the incidence increased during childhood from 1 per cent at the age of 6 years to 5 per cent at the age of 11 years. Of the migrainous children, 42 per cent were subject to one or more attacks each month which were sufficiently severe to prevent the child from carrying on with his or her usual occupation. There was no significant difference in the hours lost from school by boys with migraine than by boys who did not suffer from headache. However, migrainous girls lost a mean of 50 hours from school per term, compared with 27 hours for girls not subject to headache.

Dalsgaard-Nielson[55] reported a higher incidence than Bille for each age group in 2027 Danish children, and found that the incidence in women reached 19 per cent by the age of 40. This figure is in agreement with Waters and O'Connor[204] who calculated that 19 per cent of 2933 women between the ages of 20 and 64 years in a region of Wales suffered from migraine. Of 56 migrainous women interviewed, only 13 (23 per cent) had consulted a doctor for their headaches in the previous year and 26 (46 per cent) said that they had never seen a doctor at any time in their lives for headache.

The peak incidence of migraine is reached in women during the reproductive years of life and then declines as age advances. Whitty and Hockaday[211] obtained information about 92 patients who had attended a neurology clinic 14 years before. Attacks had ceased in 27 patients and were less severe in 44. Of the 18 patients over the age of 64 only 9 were still subject to migraine. Walker[200] studied 5785 records from a general practice in the Liverpool area of England and interviewed patients with a history of recurrent headache. A past or present history of migraine was obtained in 4·85 per cent of patients. Walker analysed the data in 150 migrainous patients over the age of 30 and found that 20 of 38 males and 84 of 112 females were subject to attacks more often than once each month. Sweetman[188] found that only one-third of the patients diagnosed as having migraine were referred to a neurologist. It is clear that migraine is a major source of morbidity in the community and is managed mainly by the general practitioner.

Definition of the Migraine Syndrome

The term migraine is of French origin and comes from the Greek 'hemicrania' like the old English word 'megrim'. The classical concept of migraine is that of a paroxysmal disturbance of cerebral function associated with unilateral headache and vomiting. The definition of migraine has widened in recent years to include bilateral headaches. It is not unusual for patients to experience pain over the entire head with the same accompaniments as their unilateral attacks. Other patients may have bilateral or unilateral headaches, which are typical of migraine in their sudden onset and severity and association with nausea and photophobia, but which are not preceded by visual or other neurological symptoms. Gowers pointed out in 1888 that the same patients may have simple headaches at one period of their life and more complex symptoms at another time.

'The simple headaches have the same characters and occur under the same causal conditions of heredity, etc., as those in which there are in addition other sensorty sympoms'.

To test the validity of this extension of the definition of migraine, a survey was done at the Northcott Neurological Centre in Sydney of 290 patients who had been diagnosed as having migraine.[166]

Classical migrainous symptoms such as aphasia, paraesthesiae and visual disturbances (ranging from flashing lights in front of the eyes through zig-zag fortification spectra to scotomas and hemianopia) occurred in 101 of these patients, preceding the headache in 49 and concurrently with the headache in 52. These cardinal symptoms of migraine were associated with bilateral headaches as often as with hemicrania. There was no significant difference in the frequency of vomiting, photophobia, scalp tenderness or other parameters of migraine between those with unilateral or bilateral headaches, and the percentage with a family history of migraine was the same in both groups. The headaches of the 189 patients who were not subject to focal neurological symptoms were otherwise typical of migraine.

The Research Group on Migraine and Headache of the World Federation of Neurology agreed on the following definition of migraine.

Migraine is a familial disorder characterized by recurrent attacks of headache widely variable in intensity, frequency and duration. Attacks are commonly unilateral and are usually associated with anorexia, nausea and vomiting. In some cases they are preceded by, or associated with, neurological and mood disturbances.

All the above characteristics are not necessarily present in each attack or in each patient. Conditions which are generally accepted as falling within the above definition are as follows:

Classical migraine, in which headache is preceded or accompanied by transient focal neurological phenomena, for example, visual, sensory or speech disturbance.

Non-classical migraine, which is not associated with sharply defined focal neurological disturbances. This is the more common variety encountered.

Conditions which may fall within the category of migraine were listed by the Research Group on Headache as follows:

Cluster headache: (Synonyms: 'Harris' ciliary or migrainous neuralgia', 'Horton's histaminic cephalgia'.) This condition is considered by the author to be an entity distinct from migraine for reasons presented in Chapter 12.

Facial migraine: (Synonym: 'lower-half headache'.) Unilateral episodic facial pain associated with symptoms suggestive either of migraine or of cluster headache.

Ophthalmoplegic migraine: Episodic migraine-like attacks associated with objective evidence of paresis of the extraocular muscles, usually those supplied by the third nerve, often outlasting the headache. A structural abnormality must be excluded before this diagnosis is made.

Hemiplegic migraine: A rare condition which may exhibit a dominant inheritance, characterized by episodic migrainous attacks associated with hemiplegia outlasting the headache.

To this list we should add the variation of 'vertebro-basilar migraine', described by Bickerstaff, in which brainstem symptoms, such as vertigo and ataxia, are associated with visual disturbance and an increased tendency to faint at the time of the migraine attack. The syndrome is thought to be caused by the constriction of the basilar and posterior cerebral arteries, and the fainting to result from ischaemia of the reticular formation.

Varieties of Migraine

The Ad Hoc Committee on Classification of Headache considered those patients with characteristic sensory, motor or visual prodromes as 'classic' migraine and those without any focal neurological disturbance as 'common' migraine.[74] This classification demarcates both ends of the spectrum but there are some patients whose headaches are difficult to classify into one group or the other because the only neurological symptoms may be vertigo, dysarthria or loss of concentration. These symptoms are almost certainly caused by the same intracranial process that is responsible for scintillating scotomas, but would not be accepted by many as criteria for 'classic migraine'. Other patients have headaches accompanied by symptoms of varying complexity so that their manifestations slide in and out of the criteria of classic migraine from episode to episode. The life history of a patient with migraine often illustrates this point. It is not uncommon for migraine to start with vomiting attacks in early childhood, to which headache may be added after some years. In later childhood the headache may become the main source of complaint and vomiting of secondary importance. As puberty is approached the classic prodromes may become superadded so that each headache is preceded by zig-zag fortification spectra or other symptoms. In middle age, vomiting may be deleted from the syndrome. At any stage of life, migrainous patients may be liable to episodes of focal neurological disturbance without headache or vomiting which are called *migraine equivalents.*

Case Report

The following illustrates a case of migraine equivalent.[166]

A university lecturer and statistician, aged 52 years, with a family history of migraine, suffered from attacks of classical migraine from the ages of 17 to 23 years. He was then free from all symptoms for 10 years, but at the age of 33 years a new symptom complex appeared without headaches. The attack would begin with sudden blurring of vision for 3 or 4 minutes followed by distressing sensations of circles, lines and zig-zags dancing in front of his eyes. The attack was accompanied by nausea, giddiness and photophobia and ceased after 30 minutes, leaving him exhausted.

In view of the wide variation in clinical symptoms, it is remarkable that there is usually little difficulty in the diagnosis of migraine, the reason being the repetitive paroxysmal nature of the disorder. Difficulty arises when the frequency of attacks is such that migraine recurs almost daily or where migraine is superimposed upon daily tension headache. In both instances it may be difficult to sort out the vascular component from the background of nervous tension or depression.

Some varieties of migraine are sufficiently distinctive to warrant consideration as separate subgroups. The pain of migraine may involve one side of the face rather than the head and the condition is then called *facial migraine* or lower-half headache.

Facial Migraine

Facial migraine is unilateral and usually starts in the palate or angle of the nose, spreads to the cheek, ear or neck, and may radiate upwards to involve the territory characteristic of cluster headache. It is distinguished from cluster headache by the longer duration of lower-half headaches, which last for more than 4 hours and may last several days, by the absence of bouts of headache alternating with periods of freedom, and by its association with typical migrainous features such as gastrointestinal disturbance. The management is essentially the same as that of migraine.

Case Report

The following is a case of lower-half headache presenting in a patient with a past history of migraine.

A woman aged 34 years had been subject to bilateral throbbing headaches, associated with nausea, vomiting, photophobia and scalp tenderness, between the ages of 3 and 20 years. These attacks recurred about twice a month and lasted for 2 days at a time. She was completely free of headache from the age of 20 years until she reached the age of

30 years, when she experienced a different kind of headache. This started in the left cheek, spread to the left ear, the angle of the jaw, and then radiated down that side of the neck. She became nauseated with the pain but did not vomit. She noticed flashes of light in front of the left eye 'like little stars' as well as tingling in the left arm, which felt unnaturally light, for half an hour at the beginning of each attack. As the pain increased, the left side of her face became puffy, the left eye watered and light hurt her eyes. The left ear ached with the headache and she heard a buzzing noise in that ear. The episodes were brought on by alcoholic drinks and relieved partly by cold compresses. Her mother and her sister suffered from typical migraine. The attacks recurred two or three times each month, lasting for 2–3 days at a time, until she was placed on methysergide 2 mg three times daily, which reduced the frequency of attacks to one in 3 months, and this attack lasted for 1 day only.

In another form, commonly running in families, unilateral weakness may be a consistent and dramatic example of focal neurological deficit accompanying migraine, and it has therefore been called *familial hemiplegic migraine*.[210] Hemiparesis is not necessarily contralateral to the side of the headache.

Case Report

The following illustrates the problem of a family with 'hemiplegic migraine'.

A man aged 49 years has been subject to bouts of numbness and paralysis of one side of the body (usually the right) since the age of 17 years, which recur every 3 months or so. He feels full of energy and in unusually good spirits for an hour or so before the attack and can then predict that one is about to start. Numbness and weakness creep up from his hand to his shoulder and then move up his leg. After half an hour the right side of his face is affected and he is unable to speak. An hour after the onset he develops a severe left-sided throbbing headache which lasts for several hours. More severe attacks are associated with vomiting, confusion and a stuporose condition which may last for several days. His father had similar attacks all his life, characterized by right-sided weakness. Two out of the patient's 6 children are affected. Peter, aged 13 years, has had 4 attacks of headache with right hemiparesis. Anthony, aged 11 years, has had 4 episodes of left-sided headache and left hemiparesis over the last 5 years.

The persistent recurrence of double vision with migraine, associated with signs of paresis of some of the muscles responsible for eye movement, has been termed *ophthalmoplegic migraine*. The third nerve is most commonly affected with the development of ptosis, a dilated pupil, and restricted movement of the eyes in all directions except lateral gaze. The condition must be distinguished from compression of the third nerve by aneurysm or other space-occupying lesion, and diagnosis can only be made after prolonged observation of the patient and exclusion of other conditions by carotid angiography.

Case Report

The following illustrates a case of ophthalmoplegic migraine.

A man aged 60 years had been subject to frequent attacks of vomiting all his childhood since the age of 2 years. In late childhood, the episodes were associated with headache behind the left eye and photophobia. From the age of 14 years, the headaches recurred at intervals of 2 weeks, the left eyelid drooped at the onset of the attack and the left pupil was seen to dilate at this time. At the age of 17 years, the left eye deviated outwards with each attack and one year later it remained permanently in the abducted position. Ptosis recurred intermittently with further headaches but persisted between attacks from the age of 19 years. He continued to have left-sided headaches once each fortnight throughout his life. One brother suffered from frequent headaches without vomiting but there was no definite family history of migraine. Apart from the left third nerve palsy, no abnormality was found on examination. No intracranial bruit could be heard. Electro-encephalography and a left carotid arteriogram were normal. His case history had been reported in 1929 by the late Dr. Eric Susman under the title of 'Migraine Ophthalmoplegique (Charcot)'.[185]

If visual hallucinations and scotomas are limited to one eye rather than one half field, then the term *retinal migraine* may be employed.

Case Report

The following illustrates a case of 'retinal migraine'.[166]

A flying instructor, aged 33 years, without a family history of migraine, developed attacks which started with a 'starry feeling' in front of the left eye. He then saw bright lights 'like silver paper' which lasted for approximately 30 seconds. Vision was then partially lost or completely lost in the left eye for a period of 5 minutes and the pupil was dilated during this time. The amblyopia then resolved, leaving a dull ache behind the left eye. He had experienced 8 attacks of this sort in a period of 2 years. Radiography of the skull, an EEG and a left carotid angiogram were normal.

If the brainstem and cerebellum are particularly affected by the vasoconstrictive phase, the syndrome is called *vertebro-basilar* migraine which will be considered further under the heading of Focal Neurological Symptoms and Signs.

Sex and Age Distribution

Migraine is much more common in women, who comprised 60 per cent of one series of 500 cases[166] and 75 per cent of another 500 cases[113] which the author had the opportunity to analyse personally. Kinnier Wilson summarized 13 published series with a total of 3278 cases of migraine and found a female preponderance of 71·6 per cent.

The first attack of migraine is experienced at the age of 10 years or younger by 25 per cent of patients (*see Figures 8.1* and *9.2*). One patient suffered his first episode at the age of 18 months. It is rare for migraine to make its appearance after the age of 45 years, but the author recalls 1 patient in whom typical migraine started at the age of 60 years. Migraine may be a lifelong complaint. The duration of headache at the time of seeking treatment in one personal series is shown in *Figure 8.2*.

Family History

When the family history includes only parents and siblings 46 per cent of migrainous patients have a family history of migraine, compared with 18 per cent of patients suffering from typical tension headache who were used as a control group.[113] If grandparents are included as well, 55 per cent of patients have a positive family history.[166] From a study of 832 offspring of 119 patients, Wolff[214] concluded that migraine was inherited, probably through a recessive gene with a penetrance of approximately 70 per cent. Some families, however, clearly illustrate a dominant inheritance.

Relationship to Epilepsy, Allergy and Childhood Vomiting Attacks

Many reports in the past have linked migraine with epilepsy, allergic disorders (asthma, hay fever, hives and eczema) and cyclical vomiting or 'bilious attacks' in childhood. Any uncontrolled observation is suspect because a migrainous patient is more likely to be referred for investigation if suffering from an associated illness, and the allergist, neurologist, psychiatrist or other specialist may receive a biased sample because of his particular interest. To obviate this, 100 patients with typical daily muscle-contraction headache were used as a control group to compare with 500 migrainous patients referred to the same clinic.[113] No significant difference in the family or personal history of epilepsy and allergy could be found between the two groups (Table 9.1). Bille[23] also found that the incidence of

97

H

allergy and epilepsy was no higher in migrainous children than in normal controls.

These observations make it clear that there is no primary relationship between migraine, epilepsy or allergy. It does not deny the possibly that allergic disturbances may trigger a migraine attack, or that the vasoconstrictive phase of migraine may precipitate epileptic phenomena in patients predisposed by their genetic constitution or a focal cortical lesion.

TABLE 9.1

PERSONAL AND FAMILY HISTORY OF MIGRAINE, EPILEPSY, ALLERGY AND VOMITING ATTACKS IN MIGRAINE AND TENSION HEADACHE

	Personal History			Family History		
	Migraine (per cent)	Tension (per cent)	Significance of difference	Migraine (per cent)	Tension (per cent)	Significance of difference
Migraine	100·0	0	Not applicable	46·0	18	P = <0·001
Epilepsy	1·6	2	Not significant	2·4	3	Not significant
Allergy	17·4	13	Not significant	8·2	6	Not significant
Childhood vomiting attacks	23·2	12	P = <0·02			

Case Report

The following illustrates a case of temporal lobe epilepsy associated with migraine.

A boy aged 16 years had been subject to 'the thing' about once a week since the age of 8 years. 'The thing' consisted of 'seeing something in my mind like a part of my past life', a sensation which lasted for less than a minute. It could represent some event well remembered or be stylized 'like a cartoon or a picture'. His words were jumbled, he could not read and wrote nonsense while the attack was upon him. About once a month 'the thing' lasted longer than usual, perhaps as long as 15 minutes on occasions, and was followed by nausea and unilateral headache which was nearly always leftsided.

He had been born of an instrumental labour and quivered down the right side shortly after birth. On examination he had a right homo-

98

nymous hemianopia. Electroencephalography disclosed a left posterior temporal sharp and slow wave focus. An air encephalogram demonstrated a porencephalic cyst which occupied the major part of the posterior quadrant of the left hemisphere (*Figure 9.1*). His temporal lobe attacks were controlled by phenytoin and carbamazepine. His migraine headaches responded to sublingual ergotamine tartrate and abated when methysergide was added to the anticonvulsant medication. The history suggests that temporal lobe epilepsy was initiated by the prodromal vasoconstrictive phase of migraine on some occasions but recurred independently at other times.

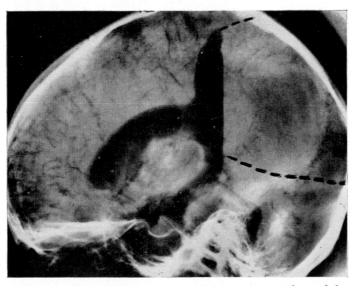

Figure 9.1. Porencephalic cyst replacing the posterior quadrant of the left cerebral hemisphere, demonstrated by pneumoencephalography. Other views taken with different head positions outlined the margins of the cyst as indicated by the interrupted lines. The patient was a boy whose attacks of temporal lobe epilepsy were often triggered by the vasoconstrictive phase of a migraine attack. (Case history in text)

In the survey, mentioned above, a past history of vomiting attacks in childhood was found significantly more frequently in migrainous patients (23 per cent) than patients with muscle-contraction headache (12 per cent), thus supporting the view that cyclical vomiting of childhood may be a precursor of adult migraine. Most children will admit to some sort of headache at the time of their vomiting attacks. Abdominal pain may accompany vomiting attacks of childhood, but cannot be regarded as a migraine equivalent if the only symptom is recurrent abdominal pain. In other words, abdominal symptoms are common in migraine, but it is doubtful whether such an entity as 'abdominal migraine' exists.

Site of Headache

Migraine headache is chiefly unilateral in two-thirds of patients and bilateral in the other third.[113] In about one-fifth of patients, the pain habitually effects the same side of the head in each attack.[166] The pain may be felt deeply behind the eye, but more commonly involves the frontal and temporal regions. It may extend over the entire head and radiate down to the face, or even to the neck and shoulders. In other patients it starts as a dull ache in the upper neck and occipital region and radiates forwards. In some patients it may remain limited to the vascular territory of frontal, temporal or occipital arteries.

Quality of Headache

Migraine commonly starts as a dull headache which rapidly becomes more severe and assumes a throbbing or pulsating quality which it may lose as the headache continues or intensifies.

Frequency of Attacks

Any analysis from a neurological clinic naturally includes patients with more frequent and severe attacks than those encountered in general practice. More than half the patients attending such a clinic experienced between one and four attacks each month (*Figure 9.3*). It is probable that emotional factors become of greater aetiological significance as the frequency of attacks increases. In the 15 per cent of patients who reported more than 10 attacks each month, tension headaches were often present as well and the patients sometimes found it difficult to distinguish the two.[166] Uncommonly patients may progress to 'status migrainosus' when they awaken each day with recrudescence of their migraine headache.

Duration of Attacks

The headache persists for less than one day in about two-thirds of patients (*Figure 9.4*), although a feeling of exhaustion and lethargy may remain for several days afterwards.

100

Time and Mode of Onset

Migraine headache may start at any time of the day, when it may be preceded by focal neurological symptoms such as visual disturbance. More commonly, the patient awakens in the early morning with the headache already present.

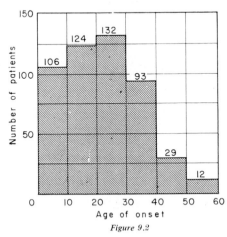

Figure 9.2

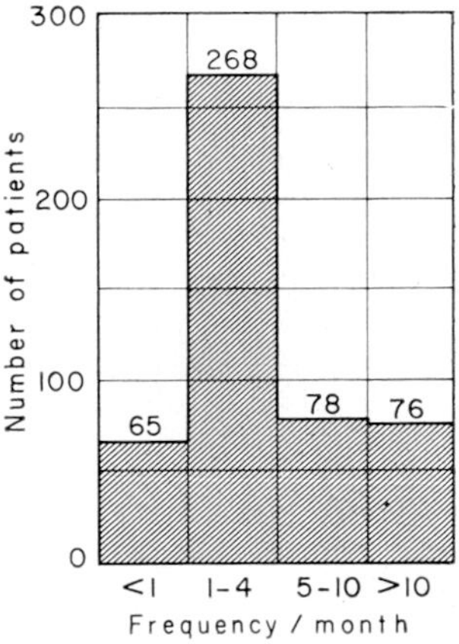

Figure 9.3

Figure 9.2. The age at which the first migraine attack occurred in the 500 patients of Selby and Lance, 1960. (This figure may be compared with that of a different series shown in Figure 8.1). (Reproduced by courtesy of the Editor of the Journal of Neurology, Neurosurgery and Psychiatry)

Figure 9.3. The frequency of migraine attacks in patients attending a neurological clinic (from Selby and Lance, 1960). (Reproduced by courtesy of the Editor of the Journal of Neurology, Neurosurgery and Psychiatry)

Figure 9.4. The customary length of each migraine headache reported by 500 patients (from Selby and Lance, 1960). (Reproduced by courtesy of the Editor of the Journal of Neurology, Neurosurgery and Psychiatry)

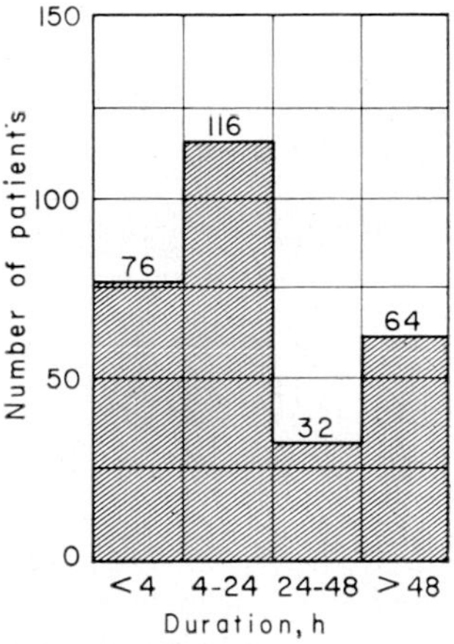

Figure 9.4

ASSOCIATED PHENOMENA

Vascular Changes

The patient with migraine often notices increased pulsation and tenderness of the superficial temporal arteries during a headache,

101

and finds that pressure over the vessel will reduce the intensity of headache. Veins may become prominent over forehead or temple and the conjunctival vessels are usually dilated. The skin may flush, but is more commonly pale and sweating in severe attacks. Hands and feet often feel cold. Patients with migraine may rarely have a fever.

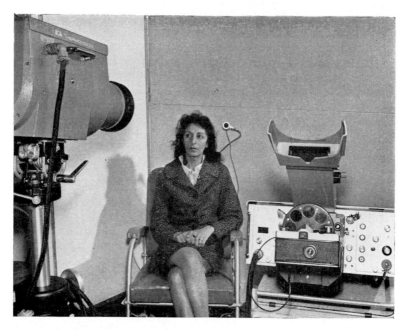

Figure 9.5. Measurement of skin temperature by the AGA thermovision camera. A temperature reference disc can be seen to the left of the patient's head. The camera is seen on the left and the viewing screen on the right

Skin Temperature

The temperature of the forehead and scalp may be measured rapidly and conveniently by means of a thermovision camera (*Figure 9.5*). This device incorporates an infra-red detector and rapid scanner and displays a picture on a television screen in which the intensity of light is proportional to skin temperature. The AGA thermovision camera is equipped to display separately each isotherm at a selected interval, such as 1 degC, and each isotherm may be photographed with a different colour filter so that the resulting picture displays the superimposed isotherms like a contour map (Plate 1). Using this device, Lance and Anthony[115] studied 15 control subjects, 10 migrainous subjects and 5 patients with cluster headache. Their experience was enlarged by study of another 100 normal subjects in a survey of cerebral vascular disease. Of the 115 normal individuals, 7 showed an asymmetrical facial thermogram. Four of these were rescreened and were then found to be normal. In contrast to this, 8 out of the 15 patients with vascular headache showed an asymmetry when free of headache, and 12 out of 15 were abnormal during a headache. Of 13 migraine headaches studied, the affected side was cooler by approximately 1 degC in 8 (Plate 1, b, c), was slightly warmer in 2, while the forehead remained symmetrical in 3. When a headache was eased by ergotamine tartrate, the temperature of the forehead became symmetrical (Plate 1, g, h). This supports the suggestion that blood is shunted away from the skin in migraine headache in spite of the dilatation of large scalp arteries.

Sodium and Fluid Retention

Increase in weight, with or without signs of generalized oedema, is noted by about one-half of migrainous patients before the migraine attack. Oliguria is common before the attack and roughly 30 per cent of patients notice polyuria as the headache subsides.[113] The blood sodium level has been shown to increase before and during headache while serum protein concentration falls.[35] The urinary output of sodium by migrainous subjects between attacks after being given a water load of 1,000–1,500 ml is almost double that of controls. There is thus evidence that sodium and fluid retention is associated with migraine, but it is unlikely to be a cause of migraine, since the administration of diuretics, which minimizes weight fluctuations, does not prevent the regular recurrence of migraine headache.[163] Stanford and Greene[184] suggested that aldosterone might be responsible for the sodium and fluid retention of migraine, and reported the cure of premenstrual migraine by the surgical treatment of Conn's syndrome.

Gastrointestinal Disturbance

About 90 per cent of patients feel nauseated with their migraine headache and the majority vomit as well. The passage of one or more loose stools at this phase of the migraine attack is noted by about 20 per cent of patients.[113] These gastrointestinal symptoms are probably not a reaction to the pain of migraine since they may occur with comparatively mild headaches, particularly in children. It is unlikely that they are caused by intracranial vasoconstriction affecting medullary centres because they are not necessarily associ-

103

ated with vertigo or other symptoms of brainstem ischaemia. Changes in plasma serotonin, described in Chapter 10, might possibly be linked with alteration of gastrointestinal motility.

Photophobia

Some 80 per cent of patients find light unpleasant during migraine headache and prefer to lie down in a darkened room. Photophobia occurs independently of conjunctival vasodilatation and may be a referred pain from irritation of the ophthalmic division of the fifth nerve.[59] Alternatively, it may be just one manifestation of hyper-activity of the special senses, since dislike of noise and strong odours are also common complaints.

Hyperaesthesia

About two-thirds of patients comment on undue sensitivity of the scalp during and after a migraine headache.[166]

FOCAL NEUROLOGICAL SYMPTOMS AND SIGNS

One of the characteristics of migraine which separates it clearly from cluster headache and, of course, from muscle-contraction headache, is its association with transient disturbance of cerebral function in about two-thirds of patients. Visual hallucinations or scotomas are most frequent, occurring in about one-third of all migrainous patients. Fortification spectra are experienced by about 10 per cent of patients, and were given this name because the zig-zag appearance of the hallucination resembles the plan of a fortified town viewed from above. The equivalent term 'teichopsia' is derived from the Greek 'teichos', meaning a wall. Another 25 per cent of patients describe unformed flashes of light ('photopsia') which are white or coloured. Symptoms which originate in areas of cortex other than the occipital lobe are much less common. Paraesthesiae around the mouth and tongue and in both hands may arise from the cortex or from the long sensory tracts in the brainstem. Strictly unilateral paraesthesiae associated with hemiparesis or dysphasia, which is clearly of cortical origin, is encountered in about 4 per cent of patients.[113] Transient temporal or parietal lobe syndromes may be part of a migraine attack. The author remembers one patient describing the distorted perception of her body image. 'My fingers felt as long as telegraph poles and my mouth with the teeth in it seemed like a cave full of tombstones.' Lewis Carroll suffered from migraine and it has been suggested that some of the inspiration for

PLATE I

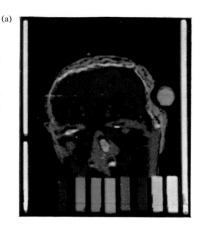

(a)

Facial thermograms in migraine and cluster headache. Each isotherm has been photographed with a different colour filter so that skin temperature may be measured by reference to the colour scale below each photograph. Each colour represents an isotherm separated by 1 degC and the green background or disc represents the reference temperature of 32°C

(a),(b),(c): Changes in migraine headache; (a) before headache, showing symmetry of forehead temperature; (b) at onset of right hemicrania showing that the right side is 1–2 degC cooler than the left; (c) at height of right hemicrania when patient is feeling nauseated. Skin temperature is a little lower but right forehead remains 1 degC cooler than the left

(d), (e): Effect of ergotamine tartrate in migraine headache; (d) patient with right-sided migraine showing that affected side is 1 degC cooler than the left; (e) after oral ergotamine, 3 mg, when headache has subsided, showing restoration of symmetry on forehead

(f)

(f), (g), (h): Changes in cluster headache; (f) before cluster headache, showing symmetry of forehead temperature; (g) early phase of cluster headache with cold patch extending over right eye on painful side; (f) later, when cold patch has disappeared and temple and cheek are warmer on the affected side. (*From Lance and Anthony, 1971*)

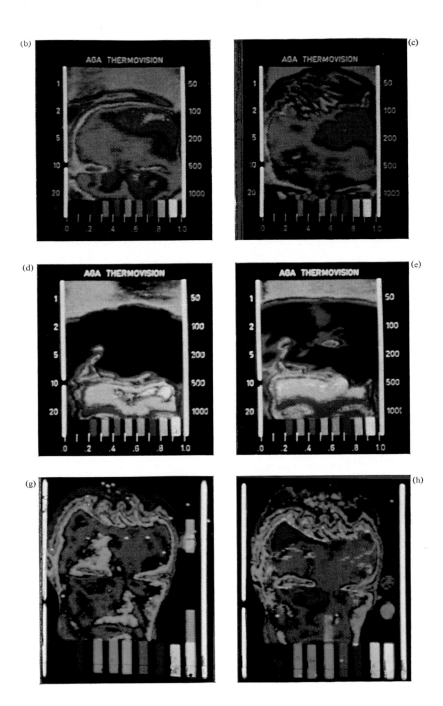

illusions of vision and body image in 'Alice in Wonderland' may have had its origin in migrainous vasospasm.

Symptoms arising from the brainstem such as diplopia, vertigo, incoordination, ataxia and dysarthria are the only neurological components of the attack in about 25 per cent of patients.[113] Bickerstaff[22] pointed out that severe brainstem symptoms in migraine were often associated with faintness, fainting or sudden loss of consciousness. He attributed this to constriction of the basilar artery which supplies the midbrain reticular formation responsible for the maintenance of consciousness. This is borne out by the experience of the author's clinic, since 7 per cent of patients with symptoms referable to the vertebrobasilar arterial system had fainted on occasions during their attacks, whereas none of those with cortical symptoms arising from areas supplied by the carotid artery had done so.[113] On the other hand, confusional states without loss of consciousness were more common in the latter group. At times behaviour may be quite bizarre at the height of a migraine head-ache, such as that of a woman who left her young child in the bath and ran aimlessly down her suburban street. The focal signs of migraine usually resolve completely after each attack but there have been reported instances of permanent visual field defect, hemiparesis or third nerve palsy after prolonged attacks. The clinical features associated with severe migraine have been analysed in detail by Klee.[106]

UNDERLYING, PRECIPITATING, AGGRAVATING AND RELIEVING FACTORS

Personality

The patient susceptible to migraine is said to be tense, meticulous and obsessional in nature. Bille[23] found that migrainous children were more anxious and sensitive than normal controls. Unfortunately there is no evidence that they are more intelligent. In an analysis of 500 migrainous patients,[166] 23 per cent exhibited obsessional trends, being unnecessarily tidy and house-proud and in the habit of double-checking their actions. Another 22 per cent were hyperactive restless individuals who found it hard to relax. Overt symptoms of anxiety in the form of tremor, nervous dyspepsia, insomnia and a tendency to overbreathe were found in another 13 per cent, one-third of whom were subject to depression at times other than their migraine attacks. Of the 500 patients, 42 per cent admitted to being 'normal'. In asking students attending lectures whether they would consider them-selves as showing similar obsessional trends or anxiety symptoms, the author has been impressed that about half the group think that they do. Possibly their less obsessional brethren do not turn up for lectures. Alternatively, migrainous patients may simply mirror the world about them.

Stress

Nervous tensions is often cited as being a cause of migraine attacks, and yet it is remarkable that many who suffer frequent attacks of migraine have no undue personal, family, occupational or financial worries. More often it is a period of relaxation after stress which may trigger off a migraine attack, exemplified by those patients who experience headache regularly on weekends when looking forward to a respite from the week's problems.

Hormonal Changes

Johannis van der Linden in *De Hemicrania Menstrua* (1666) described a unilateral headache accompanied by nausea and vomiting, recurring in the Marchioness of Brandenburg each month 'during the menstrual flux'.

The periodicity of migraine is related to the menstrual cycle in about 60 per cent of women patients, the headaches appearing just before, during or after the menses. Migraine is relieved by pregnancy in about 60 per cent of women, but this does not depend upon a previous association with menstruation, although there is a positive correlation. Of women whose migraine was linked with the menses, 64 per cent lost their headache during pregnancy, compared with 48 per cent of those in whom this relationship was absent.[113] There is no link-up between relief during pregnancy and the sex of the foetus. On the other hand, some patients may experience migraine for the first time during pregnancy. Callaghan[34] found that 20 out of 200 pregnant women had developed 'true migraine' in pregnancy, 5 who had experienced migraine before pregnancy continued to have attacks, and only 3 stated that migrainous attacks had abated with the onset of pregnancy.

This report was so at variance with common experience that Somerville[182] undertook a similar survey of 200 women attending an antenatal clinic during the last 4 weeks of pregnancy. He found that 31 patients had been subject to migraine headache in the 12 months before becoming pregnant, giving an incidence of 15 per cent for women in the reproductive years. Of the 31 patients, 24 improved during pregnancy, 7 becoming completely free of headache. Only 7 patients had developed migraine for the first time in the current pregnancy, mostly in the first trimester. Somerville found that there was no significant difference in the plasma progesterone of those women whose migraine had improved (98·4 ng/ml), those women whose migraine continued during pregnancy (101·2 ng/ml) and the non-migrainous control patients (119·4 ng/ml).

Over the past few years, Somerville has clarified the relationship of migraine to the hormonal changes of the menstrual cycle in a series of important papers.[179,180,181] Normal and migrainous

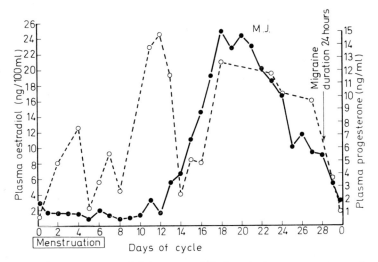

Figure 9.6. Plasma oestradiol (interrupted line) and plasma progesterone (continuous line) estimated daily during a normal menstrual cycle. Premenstrual migraine occurs during the falling phase of both curves (from Somerville, 1972,[181] by courtesy of the editor of 'Neurology')

women were found to have a similar fluctuation of hormonal levels. Plasma oestradiol rose to an early preovulatory peak, followed by a rapid fall, then a secondary rise during the luteal phase with a final fall before menstruation (Figure 9.6). Plasma progesterone remained low during menstruation and the follicular phase, then increased at or just after mid-cycle to a plateau during the luteal phase, then declined premenstrually. There was no significant difference between the peak progesterone concentrations in migrainous and non-migrainous women. Premenstrual migraine occurred regularly during or after plasma oestradiol and progesterone fell to their lowest levels. To determine which of these hormones was the more influential in triggering migraine headache,

Somerville treated 6 women with progesterone and 6 women with oestradiol in the premenstrual phase while measuring their hormonal levels daily. He found that the administration of progesterone to maintain artificially high blood levels postponed uterine bleeding,

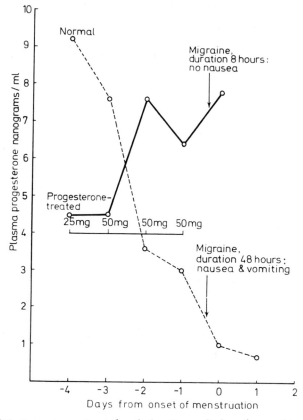

Figure 9.7. Progesterone-treated cycle (continuous line) and normal cycle (interrupted line) in the same patient. Migraine occurs at the usual time in spite of high blood levels of progesterone (from Somerville, 1971,[180] by courtesy of the editor of 'Neurology')

but that the migraine attack occurred in 5 of the 6 women at the anticipated time in the cycle (*Figure 9.7*). On the other hand, the injection of oestradiol did not postpone menstruation but delayed the onset of migraine headache in all patients by 3–9 days (*Figure 9.8*). Migraine began after the oestradiol level fell below 20 ng/100 ml and could not be postponed further if another injection of oestradiol

108

was given at this time. Two other women had consistently low levels of progesterone indicating the absence of ovulation. One developed migraine 10 days after an injection of oestradiol, followed on the eleventh day by oestrogen-withdrawal bleeding. The second patient, who was menopausal, suffered a typical episode of migraine as the oestrogen level fell 9 days after injection, without any withdrawal bleeding.

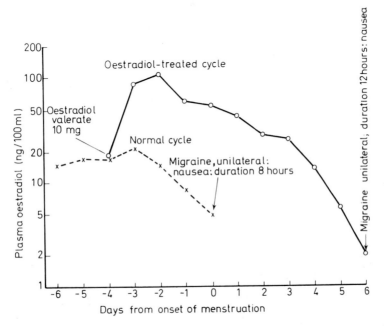

Figure 9.8. Oestrogen-treated cycle (continuous line) and normal cycle (interrupted line) in the same patient. The onset of migraine is postponed until the oestrogen level falls (from Somerville, 1972,[181] by courtesy of the editor of 'Neurology')

It is therefore apparent that the withdrawal of oestrogen, rather than progesterone, sets in motion a series of changes which culminate in the onset of migraine. This could account for the mid-cycle headache which afflicts some women in addition to menstrual migraine. There is probably some intermediary between oestrogen withdrawal and the sequelae of menstruation and migraine. The prostaglandins are possible contenders because of their actions on the uterus, and the known effect of PGE_1 in precipitating migraine when infused into normal subjects.[36]

The use of oral contraceptive tablets commonly exacerbates migraine,[151,212] and permanent neurological deficit has been reported in patients whose phase of intracranial vasoconstriction was prolonged while taking oral contraceptives.[78] Progestogenic agents have been advocated in the treatment of migraine[128] but a comparative study from Newcastle upon Tyne showed that this method of treatment is less effective than the use of methysergide[95] although a later trial by the same group did demonstrate superiority of flumedroxone (Demigran) over placebo. An unpublished trial of allyloestrenol in 20 patients from our clinic was not encouraging, and more recently Somerville and Carey used a constant contraceptive dose of the new synthetic progestogen, 3-acetoxychlormadinone, to suppress ovulation, with improvement in some 40 per cent of patients. The use of progestogenic agents is complicated by a high incidence of menstrual disturbances and does not seem to be worth pursuing at the moment, particularly in view of the implication of oestrogens as the more important trigger factor.

Foods and Eating Habits

About 25 per cent of patients consider that their attacks are provoked by eating certain foods, particularly fatty foods, chocolates and oranges.[166] Tomatoes, onions and pineapples are occasionally mentioned. There is some doubt whether this is an idiosyncrasy or an allergic response, or whether it depends on a conditioned reflex. Wolff[214] quotes experiments in which incriminated foods were ingested by patients without their knowledge and without a headache ensuing. On the other hand the giving of capsules containing an inert substance with the suggestion that they contained chocolate or other offending food was often followed by an episode of migraine.

Recently tyramine 100 mg has been reported as producing migraine headache in patients who considered that dietary factors influenced their attacks, whereas lactose in identical capsules did not.[85] It is possible that certain foods contain amines which may be responsible for a sequence of biochemical changes when absorbed. Tyramine, for example, may play a part in the release of serotonin from platelets, which is discussed in Chapter 10. There is evidence that those patients who experience migraine after the ingestion of tyramine have a defect in enzyme inactivation which allows sufficient free tyramine to enter the blood stream and initiate a further sequence of events with headache as the end-point.[162b]

Missing a meal may sometimes precipitate migraine, possibly because of a lowered level of blood sugar,[24] which may in turn stimulate the production of noradrenaline and other biochemical changes. The level of free fatty acids in the blood increases more in those fasting patients who develop migraine than those who do not.[93]

Glare and Noise

Approximately one-half of patients state that glare will precipitate headache. This includes watching moving pictures or television as well as spending a sunny day at the beach. Noise is also implicated by some patients.

Vasodilatation

Alcohol and other vasodilators are well recognized as inducers of migraine or cluster headache and vasocontrictor drugs are instrumental in ending it.

Exertion may provoke a migraine attack or other varieties of vascular headache. Pressure over dilated scalp arteries or the application of cold packs will often relieve the headache. The reason for hot packs relieving some patients' attacks is less obvious but could be that capillary vasodilatation reduces the internal pressure and hence the distension of larger proximal vessels.

Associated Diseases

Migraine may be aggravated by hypertension[200] and aldosteronism.[184] It has been reported as a symptom of hyper-pre-bcta lipoproteinacmia, possibly because of changes in plasma viscosity or red cell aggregation, and disappears with restoration of serum lipids to normal.[125] There is still some dispute as to the significance of cervical spondylosis and whether compression of the vertebral arteries or their sympathetic plexus by osteophytes can give rise to 'migraine cervicale'.

PHYSICAL EXAMINATION

There are no physical signs of migraine detectable between attacks. Hearing a bruit over the skull or orbits may give rise to concern and warrant carotid angiography to exclude the presence of an intracranial aneurysm or angioma. In one series of 500 patients, 10 were found to have an audible cranial bruit.[166] Two were children under the age of 10 years in whom skull bruits are usually not of any significance. In 4 adult patients the bruit was heard over both eyes, and in 4 it was unilateral. Carotid angiograms in 3 of the latter were completely normal.

In the above-mentioned series, a blood pressure of more than 150 mm systolic and 100 mm diastolic was found in 13 per cent of patients. Hypertension is said to be significantly more common over the age of 50 years in migrainous patients than the general population.[200]

While a migraine headache is in progress, excessive pulsation of temporal arteries may be noted and veins are often prominent on forehead and temple. The face and scalp are commonly pale and sweaty in severe attacks. The patient may be mentally confused, stuporose or even lose consciousness for a brief time. Speech may be slurred (dysarthria) or there may be inability to choose the correct word or phrase (dysphasia). There may be a transient Horner's syndrome or paresis of the third cranial nerve. More rarely, hemi-paresis or involuntary movements may be observed at the height of the attack. The patient may be ataxic and have difficulty with co-ordination. Such patients of mine have been suspected of drunken-ness and questioned by the police when struggling to get home after being taken unawares by a migraine attack. They now carry a letter explaining the vagaries of migraine.

10—The Pathogenesis of Migraine

Headache, which is one of the most serious complaints, is sometimes occasioned by an intemperament solely; sometimes by a redundance of humours, and sometimes by both . . .

Paul of Aegina, circa A.D. 600
(Tr. Adams, 1844)[3]

THE MECHANISM OF PAIN PRODUCTION IN MIGRAINE HEADACHE

The pain of migraine was long suspected to be of vascular origin because of the observation that arteries and veins were prominent in the forehead and temples during the attack and that pressure over the scalp vessels or the common carotid artery in the neck eased the pain to some extent. In 1938, Graham and Wolff published an important paper showing that the amplitude of pulsation of scalp arteries increased with the onset of migraine and correlated well with the severity of the headache at each stage of the attack.[81] The injection of ergotamine tartrate reduced the pulsation of the extracranial arteries by 50 per cent at the same time as the headache was relieved. Graham and Wolff recorded the pulsation of the CSF as an indirect method of measuring dilatation of intracranial vessels and found that there was no increase during migraine headache or any significant reduction after the injection of ergotamine tartrate. However, there is some doubt about the accuracy with which the CSF pulse reflects changes in calibre of intracranial vessels, since it has been shown that spinal arteries make a major contribution to the pulse wave, at least in the dog. Other evidence that migraine headache was caused by arteries of the scalp rather than those inside the skull came from comparisons with histamine headache which had been studied by Pickering and Hess in 1933.[150] The intravenous infusion of histamine causes flushing followed by headache which comes on after the scalp arteries have returned to their normal calibre,[199] whereas CSF pulsation is still increased by 250 per cent while histamine headache is in progress.[81] Increasing intracranial pressure to 1000 mm CSF relieves histamine headache immediately

113

but has no effect on the headache of migraine.[164] It may be concluded that dilatation of intracranial vessels is responsible for the headache caused by histamine, but not that of migraine. Irrespective of their contribution to headache, the intracranial vessels are thought to dilate in some migraine attacks. On one occasion a burr-hole exploration was done at the height of migraine headache and a tight, non-pulsating dura was found. The brain looked oedematous and cerebral blood vessels were seen to be dilated.[79]

Further evidence about the vascular nature of migraine, although not discriminating between the part played by intracranial and extracranial arteries, was brought forward by Wolff,[214] who spun patients in a human centrifuge at a positive acceleration of 2·0 G. with a complete relief of headache. It is a pity that this treatment is impractical as an office procedure.

Thus the evidence has slowly accumulated that migraine is of vascular origin and that it is chiefly the extracranial arteries which are at fault. Artificial distension of one superficial temporal artery will reproduce the pain of migraine in the temple.[153]. It has been shown that the pulsation of the superficial temporal artery is larger than normal in migrainous subjects, even at times of freedom from headache, and that it becomes more variable 3–4 days before a headache.[196] Just before an attack, while a patient is experiencing the phase of visual scotomas, the amplitude of pulsation is at its lowest. As the headache develops, the pulsation increases on the affected side.[195] Conjunctival vessels may dilate on the side of headache and become less sensitive to the local application of vasoconstrictor agents such as noradrenaline.[146] Blau and Davis[25] have recently reported that the conjunctival vessels constricted in half the patients observed and dilated in the remainder. The changes were bilateral although more evident on the side of headache, and intravascular red cell aggregation was seen in all cases. Tissue clearance studies using radioactive sodium have shown that skin blood flow increases in the fronto-temporal region during migraine, more so on the side of the headache.[63]

These observations make it clear that the scalp arteries dilate and cause headache in migraine. How can this be so, when no normal person experiences headache after strenuous exercise or a hot shower or bath which causes obvious dilatation of scalp vessels? One explanation is that dilatation of the capillaries does not keep pace with the arteries in migraine, so that the vessel wall becomes overdistended. There is an analogous situation when cold is applied to the forehead of normal persons. The small vessels constrict in response to cold while the large vessels are still dilated; the subject

114

feels pain at this stage, although the pain is not really the same as that of migraine.[89] This concept of imbalance between the calibre of large and small vessels is supported by the appearance of most patients who look pale during migraine headache in spite of their bounding temporal pulses. Skin temperature is lower on the affected side of the head in the majority of migrainous patients[115] (Plate 1). Lund[127] has claimed that the administration of substances which dilate small vessels relieves migraine headache and restores the shape of the arterial pulse wave to normal, even though the amplitude remains constant at its former high level. It is hard to reconcile this idea with the knowledge that skin blood flow (measured by injected isotopes) is increased during migraine.[63] Possibly shunting of blood may take place deep to the constricted skin capillaries, thus removing injected isotope rapidly, while an increased pressure is sustained in the major scalp arteries. Heyck[90] found that the arteriovenous oxygen saturation difference between arterial blood and venous blood from the external jugular vein (mean 4·8 vol. per cent) was normally less than that between arterial blood and the cubital vein (mean 8·75 vol. per cent) but fell to a mean of 1·5 vol. per cent on the side of headache during a migraine attack and to 3·5 vol. per cent on the relatively painless side. After migraine had abated, the value on the previously affected side had returned to 4·15 vol. per cent in the 6 patients studied. This indicates that scalp blood flow is greater than that of the arm relative to its metabolic requirements and suggests that flow is augmented in the scalp during migraine headache, even though the skin capillaries are constricted.

An important factor in the production of pain from migrainous vessels appears to be the accumulation around the dilated arteries of various substances which are capable of sensitizing them to pain. A polypeptide has been found in the periarterial fluid sampled during migraine headache which is similar to the polypeptide found in blister fluid. Wolff and his colleagues called this substance 'neurokinin' and thought that it could be responsible for setting up a sterile inflammatory response in the vessel.[39,144] They considered that biopsies of the scalp arteries taken at the time of headache showed pallor and homogenous staining of the perivascular tissue which suggested that the vessel wall was oedematous.[144] These changes are equivocal and recent observers have not agreed that there is any definite abnormality.[1] However, the presence of 'neurokinin' has to be considered in discussing the mechanism of migraine, since it is known to be a potent pain-provoking substance like bradykinin. Sictueri[168] has reported that mast cells are reduced in number and in granulation, in biopsy specimens taken at the time of headache.

Thonnard-Neumann and Taylor[194] found that the number of basophil leucocytes in blood taken from an ear-lobe on the side of headache was increased in comparison with the headache-free side, although this may be a non-specific reaction to vasodilatation (Appenzeller, unpublished observations). The basophil cells on the affected side were degranulated.[193] The local release of heparin and histamine from mast and basophil cells may be associated with the accumulation of kinins in the vessel wall and possibly with the local action of serotonin in the production of pain from distended arteries during migraine.

Enough evidence has been brought forward now to make it clear that the control of extracranial blood vessels must be faulty in migraine. Histological studies have shown that the vascular pattern in some other parts of the body is abnormal in migrainous patients. Capillary loops in the nail bed and mucous membrane of the lip are of immature appearance in the majority of migraine patients,[88,154] and unusual groups of arterioles have been found in endometrial biopsies of migrainous women.[82] There are no similar observations on the vascular pattern on the scalp which would be of more direct relevance to the problem we are considering.

THE CAUSE OF FOCAL NEUROLOGICAL SYMPTOMS IN MIGRAINE

Neurological symptoms are experienced by about 65 per cent of patients, either preceding or during migraine headache. One-third of patients complain of visual disturbance; 4 per cent notice other cortical symptoms such as aphasia and unilateral paraesthesiae; and one-quarter have vertigo, slurred speech or other brainstem symptoms.[113] Such symptoms may appear transiently and inconstantly or may regularly develop over 10–30 minutes, suggesting a slow march of inhibition moving over the cerebral cortex.

Goltman had the unusual opportunity of observing a patient with a frontal skull defect while a migraine attack was in progress.[79] The scalp was depressed at the site of the skull defect when the headache began, but filled up as pain spread over the head until there was a bulging, non-pulsatile mass palpable at the height of the headache, which subsided as the headache wore off. This sequence suggests that a phase of cerebral vasoconstriction was followed by vasodilatation and cerebral oedema. The large cerebral arteries do not usually constrict since the majority of angiograms taken during an attack have been completely normal.[32] Cerebral angiography may be normal in spite of the presence of gross neurological deficit in the prodromal phase of migraine, at a time when blood flow is reduced by 50 per cent in the appropriate brain areas.[177] Skinhøj,[177] using the technique of intracarotid injection of radioactive xenon, also demonstrated that blood flow increases by 50 per cent at the height of headache. These observations support those of O'Brien,[139] who found a reduction of cortical perfusion of 20 per cent during the prodromal phase and an increase during the stage of headache, using radioactive xenon by inhalation. Constriction of retinal vessels has been described in patients with unilateral impairment of vision as a prodrome of migraine, and such defects may become permanent as the result of thrombosis of the central retinal artery or its branches.[37] Damage to the cerebral hemispheres or brainstem may also result from migraine, presumably as a result of prolonged vasospasm.

Local changes have been recorded in the electroencephalogram from the back of the scalp overlying the visual cortex during the prodromal symptoms of migraine, with focal slow waves appearing over the left occipital region when visual hallucinations were noticed in the right half-field and vice versa. A number of observations have been made on servicemen exposed to simulated high altitudes in a low-pressure chamber,[65] or simulated depths of diving in a high-pressure chamber.[6] Restoration of the barometric pressure to normal triggered migraine attacks in susceptible people and also produced visual episodes in some who had never experienced migraine before. The EEG focus resolved as the symptoms disappeared.

Pre-headache scotomas may be induced by the intravenous infusion of the vasoconstrictor agent noradrenaline and can be relieved in some patients by the use of vasodilators such as amyl nitrite or the inhalation of 10 per cent carbon dioxide in air or oxygen which has a potent effect in dilating intracranial arteries.[214]

These observations all imply that vasoconstriction is important in the genesis of neurological symptoms in migraine but there may be other factors as well. Neurophysiologists recognize a curious reaction called 'spreading depression' which takes place in animal brain when it has been damaged by dehydration or hypoxia.[130] Waves of inhibition move slowly over the cerebral cortex, preventing normal activity. Lashley[123] plotted the expansion of his own visual scotoma in migraine and calculated that the visual cortex was being suppressed by some process advancing at the rate of about 3 mm each minute. This is the same rate of progress as the 'spreading depression' which interferes with cortical recordings in animal experiments.[137] Spreading depression is associated with dilatation of the pial arteries and cerebral oedema but may be preceded by a phase of vasoconstriction.[130] It is tempting to postulate that the vasoconstrictor phase of migraine triggers off the ionic changes responsible for 'spreading depression' which thus causes the slow march of neurological symptoms in migraine.[18]

The third nerve may be temporarily paralysed in some migraine attacks (ophthalmoplegic migraine) and the mechanism is probably different from that of other symptoms and signs. Wolff has suggested that the third nerve may be compressed by dilated arteries as it passes between the posterior cerebral and superior cerebellar arteries, or that oedema of one cerebral hemisphere may be sufficient to force part of the temporal lobe into the tentorial notch, thus stretching the third nerve.[214]

DISORDERED VASCULAR CONTROL IN MIGRAINE

The sympathetic nervous system does exercise some control over intracerebral vessels but from all accounts this is weak, inconsistent and without tonic effect. Stimulation of the cervical sympathetic trunk has produced a mild constriction of the pial arteries in some recorded animal experiments, although this is not invariable. Blood flow in the internal carotid artery of the monkey has been shown to decrease by about 30 per cent.[135] However, section of the cervical sympathetic does not increase cerebral blood flow or oxygen availability in cat or monkey,[135] suggesting that the sympathetic nervous system is not responsible for maintaining vasomotor tone. This is consistent with observations in man that stellate ganglion blockade, unilateral or bilateral, does not augment cerebral blood flow.

The effect of sympathetic stimulation is greater on extracranial vessels, causing a decrease in oxygen availability in the temporalis muscle in cat and monkey, and reducing blood flow in the monkey external carotid by about 68 per cent.[135] It is doubtful whether this action has any physiological significance since the forehead and scalp are not susceptible to the sort of vasoconstrictor reflexes that are seen in the hands and feet. Startle, immersion of the hand in iced water, or taking a deep breath do not affect pulsation in forehead skin. The vascular reactions of the forehead are like those of a sympathectomized digit in that constriction is gradual as skin temperature falls, probably because of the direct effect of cold on the vessels.[89] Heat loss from the forehead remains constant during body cooling while heat loss from the fingers decreases by a factor of six.[77] Unilateral cervicodorsal ganglionectomy results in a consistent rise in skin temperature in the limbs, but not in the face or scalp. Blocking the cervical sympathetic in three subjects, of whom the author was one, did not increase the amplitude of pulsation of the superficial temporal artery. There is little increase in heat flow after blockade of scalp nerves.[71]

It is therefore evident that the sympathetic nervous system plays little part in maintaining tonic constriction of scalp vessels. On the other hand, it is known to be important in vasodilator reflexes. Capillary dilator fibres pass from the anterior thoraco-lumbar nerve roots and sympathetic ganglia and are distributed to vessels of the scalp and forehead. There is evidence that some vasodilator fibres pass out in the trigeminal nerve.[140] Blushing is abolished by sympathectomy, and flushing of the scalp and forehead no longer occurs in response to overheating of the body after sympathectomy or blockade of the cutaneous nerve supply to those areas.[71]

When skin of the trunk or legs is heated, forearm vessels dilate reflexly in normal subjects. Appenzeller and his colleagues[13] found that this response was reduced or absent in 8 out of 10 migrainous patients, but this has not been confirmed by more recent experiments.[73,92,129] There have been no comparable observations on the reactions of scalp vessels, which is a pity because they are more pertinent to the problem of migraine. When a migrainous patient stands suddenly, the pulsation of scalp arteries diminishes, unlike those of normal subjects, suggesting that there might be some defect in vasomotor control.[207] The adventitial collagen around migrainous arteries absorbs noradrenaline more than that of normal subjects when incubated with noradrenaline.[1] This may be a primary change in the adventitia or be a reaction to repeated dilatation of the vessels.

There is a small parasympathetic contribution to the carotid plexus from the greater superficial petrosal nerve, a branch of the facial nerve. Stimulation of the facial nerve results in slight and inconstant dilatation of pial blood vessels.[42] Internal carotid blood flow increases only if systemic blood pressure increases, and thus appears to be a passive effect.[135]

Many early reports on the effect of surgical procedures in migraine are invalidated by doubtful diagnosis and inadequate follow-up. It is clear that cervical sympathectomy does not provide any lasting benefit in migraine,[159,208] and section of the greater superficial petrosal nerve does not prevent migraine.[159] Ligation of the external carotid artery or the middle meningeal artery, or both, is unreliable in its effects.[141] Removal of the carotid body on the appropriate side cannot be recommended in the treatment of migraine.[118] The only operation which is of predictable benefit is that of section of trigeminal pathways, which gives relief from pain at the expense of permanent facial analgesia.[141,149,159]

It may be concluded that there is no convincing evidence at present that the neural control of blood vessels is impaired in migraine, that migraine is caused by an abnormal neural discharge, or that operation on nerve pathways will prevent migraine.

The Possibility of Defective Humoral Control of Cranial Vessels in Migraine

If the vascular changes of migraine are not caused by abnormal neural discharge, can they be explained by changes in chemical vasomotor regulation? Many vasoactive substances are contained in blood, some within the formed elements (such as histamine in leucocytes, or serotonin in platelets) and some free in the plasma.

Acetylcholine

Acetylcholine causes vasodilatation by relaxing arterioles, and the conjunctival vessels become particularly sensitive to its action during migraine headache.[144] Kunkle[107] found that acetylcholine was present in CSF samples of 4 out of 14 patients with cluster headache, in one patient with atypical migraine, but not in 7 patients with typical migraine. Migraine cannot be induced by injection of acetylcholine or metacholine.[143] There is thus no evidence at the moment to implicate acetylcholine in migraine.

Histamine

Histamine relaxes capillaries although it may constrict arteries and arterioles. Infusion of histamine produces headache by causing intracranial vascular dilatation.[150] A histamine liberating substance, compound 48/80, will release histamine from tissue stores and cause headache.[173] As mentioned earlier in this chapter, the characteristics of histamine headache are quite different from migraine.[164] Antihistamines will prevent histamine headache but are ineffective in migraine.[144] A slight increase in blood histamine can be detected at the conclusion of a migraine headache, which contrasts with the sharp rise found in cluster headache.[11] It appears unlikely that histamine plays any primary role in the pathophysiology of migraine.

Bradykinin

Bradykinin is a nonapeptide which has a vasodilator and hypotensive action. It is released from an inactive alpha 2-globulin precursor, kininogen, by proteolytic enzymes in the blood, the plasma kallikreins. It has been reported that plasma kininogen is diminished at the end of the migraine attack and that a bradykinin-releasing enzyme is increased at the time of headache.[168] The injection of bradykinin into arteries causes pain.[170] The pain-provoking action of bradykinin is potentiated by serotonin,[169] and it is possible that the local accumulation of these and allied substances may play a part in the production of vascular pain. The intradermal injection of bradykinin into the temporal area causes transient local pain but does not reproduce vascular headache.[63] The intra-venous infusion of bradykinin in man does not cause headache.[72] The flushing attacks of some cases of carcinoid tumour and the dumping syndrome are caused by increase in circulating bradykinin, but are not associated with headache. It therefore seems unlikely that bradykinin plays a primary role in migraine.

Noradrenaline

Noradrenaline constricts arterioles and capillaries in the con-junctiva. The sensitivity of these vessels to the topical application of noradrenaline increases in the phase of visual disturbance pre-ceding migraine and diminishes during headache.[146] Wolff gave intravenous infusions of noradrenaline to migrainous patients at a rate sufficient to cause contraction of the conjunctival vessels and reduce pulsation of the extracranial arteries. When the infusion took place at the height of headache, the headache usually diminished and gradually disappeared. When noradrenaline was infused in headache-free periods for up to 3 hours and then stopped, no head-ache ensued, showing that migraine headache is not simply a rebound phenomenon following tissue ischaemia.[214]

Evidence that noradrenaline is involved in the mechanism of migraine is, to date, scanty. There have been conflicting reports about the urinary excretion of one of the important catabolites of noradrenaline, vanilmandelic acid (VMA, 4-hydroxy-3-methoxy-mandelic acid). Two groups of experimenters have found an increased excretion of VMA during migraine headache[46,167] but another group dissents.[50] The question of the part played by noradrenaline in migraine must remain open. In a preliminary study of 10 patients, Dr. Hinterberger in our laboratory has not found any significant difference in adrenaline or noradrenaline levels in blood or urine in migraine.

Another vasoconstrictor substance has been found in the rabbit which has been called SVPx (substance for vasoconstriction from plasma).[216] In the rabbit, noradrenaline and adrenaline are not found in sufficient concentration to contract vascular smooth muscle and histamine exerts only a modest contracting effect. Serotonin and SVPx appear to be the two important naturally occurring vaso-constrictors in the rabbit, and it remains to be seen whether SVPx is of significance in man.

Serotonin

Serotonin constricts large arteries and veins and dilates arterioles and capillaries, but the effect varies in different species and depends, in the case of small vessels, on the degree of pre-existing neurogenic vascular tone. Since the nervous system does not con-tribute much to the maintenance of tone in cranial vessels, the latter point need not concern us here.

The direct application of serotonin to the exposed cortex con-stricts the large cerebral vessels in man as well as in the cat.[8] The intravenous injection of serotonin causes blanching of the exposed cerebral cortex in dogs and cats. The injection of serotonin into the carotid artery causes constriction of the large cerebral arteries in the monkey and slightly reduces the calibre of cerebral arteries in man. Human extracranial arteries constrict strongly after serotonin is injected into the common carotid artery and the effect persists for up to 8 minutes (*Figure 10.1*). Grimson *et al*[83] found that flow in the external carotid artery of baboons increased during the intracarotid infusion of serotonin. However, preliminary work by Welch and Spira in our laboratory has shown that flow in the external carotid artery of the monkey consistently diminishes in response to serotonin. Unpublished studies by Glover and Somerville have demonstrated that serotonin is a potent constrictor of human temporal arteries removed at autopsy and examined *in vitro*.

The main breakdown product of serotonin, 5-hydroxyindoleacetic acid (5HIAA) is excreted in excess in the urine of some patients during migraine headache (*Figure 10.2*).[46,50,174] The urinary con-centration of 5HIAA also increases, indicating that the changes cannot be explained by the polyuria which frequently accompanies migraine.[46]

There is considerable diurnal and individual variation in blood serotonin levels, so that random sampling is meaningless. Once a baseline has been established for each patient, a slight rise in plasma serotonin may be seen at the onset of a migraine attack and then the level falls sharply with the onset of headache[7,45,46] (*Figures 10.3 and 10.4*). Plasma serotonin tends to increase after vomiting or diarrhoea takes place during the headache but the effect is inconsistent. Serotonin levels do not change in cluster headache or when a head-

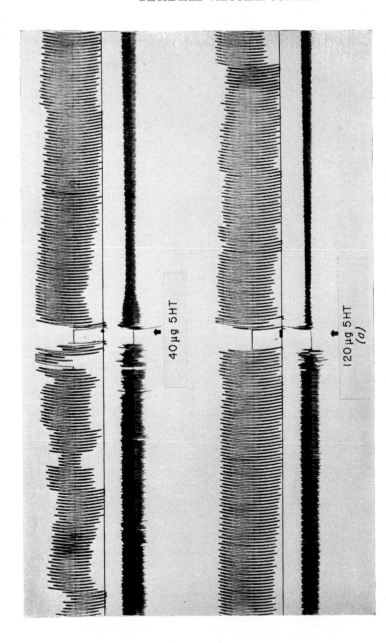

Figure 10.1. Constriction of scalp arteries induced by the intracaroid injection of serotonin. The upper trace in each instance is a recording of respiratory excursion and the lower shows the amplitude of pulsation in the superficial temporal artery. It can be seen that the intracarotid injection of 40 μg serotonin produced mild vasoconstriction and that the effect was more pronounced with 120 μg serotonin. The injection of normal saline did not alter the tracing. (From Lance, Anthony and Gonski (1967). Reproduced by courtesy of the editor of 'Archives of Neurology')

123

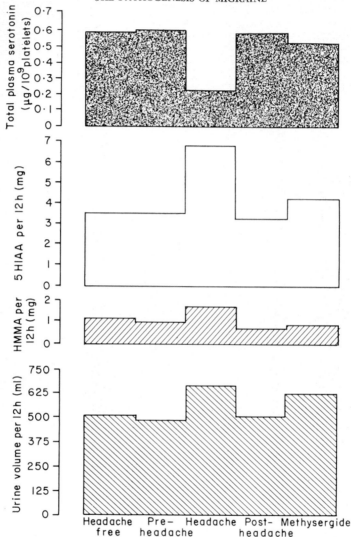

Figure 10.2. Metabolic changes in migraine. Representation of mean values for plasma serotonin; the urinary excretion of the catabolite of serotonin, 5-hydroxyindoleacetic acid (5HIAA); the urinary excretion of the catabolite of noradrenaline, 4-hydroxy-3-methoxymandelic acid (HMMA, VMA); and urine volume before, during and after a migraine headache, and during the first 24 hours of methysergide therapy. It can be seen that plasma serotonin drops in migraine headache, as 5HIAA and HMMA excretion rises. (From Curran, Hinterberger and Lance, (1967). Reproduced by courtesy of the Publishers of 'Research and Clinical Studies in Headache')

ache is induced by air encephalography, even when it is quite as severe as that of migraine and gives rise to nausea and vomiting. Other stressful procedures such as arteriography, gastroscopy and bronchoscopy do not alter the serotonin levels.[7] It is thus apparent that the fall in plasma serotonin is specific for migraine headache and not a general response to any form of headache, pain or stress.

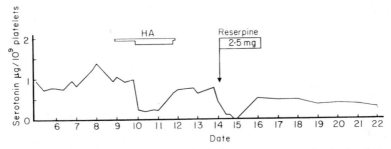

Figure 10.3. Changes in plasma serotonin during a spontaneous migraine headache, and following the injection of reserpine. The unfilled bar labelled HA marks the time of headache, the initial slender portion indicating a premonitory sensation of 'heaviness' in the head (from Anthony, Hinterberger and Lance (1967). Reproduced by courtesy of the editor of 'Archives of Neurology')

Serotonin is carried in the blood almost entirely by the platelets. The platelets retain their normal content of adenine nucleotides, adenosine triphosphate (ATP), diphosphate (ADP) and monophosphate (AMP) during migraine and are capable of taking up serotonin in normal amounts when incubated with excess.[8] The factor responsible for the loss of serotonin in migraine is found in the plasma. Plasma from specimens taken during migraine is capable of releasing serotonin when incubated with platelets from headache-free periods. The final level of serotonin in the platelet after incubation is remarkably similar to that estimated in the original blood specimen collected during the headaches.[8] The nature of this 'serotonin-releasing factor' is unknown at present. Cortisone and hydrocortisone are capable of preventing the uptake of serotonin by platelets but no substantial changes in plasma 11-oxysteroids have been found during the migraine attack.[8] Serum tryptic (arginyl-esterase) activity has also been examined without any consistent variation being demonstrated.[8] Possibilities not yet examined include other proteolytic enzymes, fatty acids, amines such as tyramine or tryptamine, and the products of antigen–antibody reactions. The demonstration that the intravenous infusion of prostaglandin E_1 will evoke headache,[36] which may be unilateral and accompanied by nausea, abdominal pain and visual disturbance in subjects who have never experienced migraine, arouses speculation about the serotonin-releasing activity of this lipid-soluble hydroxy acid.

The intramuscular injection of reserpine lowers plasma serotonin. At the same time normal subjects experience a dull headache, and the majority of migrainous patients undergo a typical migraine headache. Curzon, Barrie and Wilkinson[49] found that 5 HIAA and VMA excretion was increased 4–8 hours after the injection of reserpine in 9 out of 16 patients who developed migraine. This 4-hour period of enhanced excretion may have been missed by Tandon, Sur and Nath[191] who could not demonstrate any change in 24-hour specimens collected after the injection of reserpine. The intravenous injection of serotonin 2–7·5 mg in spontaneous or reserpine-induced migraine increases plasma serotonin and alleviates the headache (*Table 10.1*).[7,104]

TABLE 10.1

Summary of changes in Mean Total Plasma Serotonin
($\mu g/10^9$ platelets)

	No. of patients	Before	After
Onset of migraine	21	0·82	0·45
Stressful Procedures	9	0·81	0·81
Vomiting during Headache	12	0·39	0·45
Injected Reserpine 2·5 mg	13	0·75	0·35
Injected Serotonin 2–7·5 mg	6	0·37	0·52

Serotonin does not pass readily through the blood-brain barrier and its concentration in the cerebrospinal fluid is unaltered in migraine headache.[17,183] The peri-arterial injection of serotonin sometimes produces a low-grade headache extending from the point of injection over the same side of the head,[144] but on other occasions no headache ensues.[104] Serotonin reduces glomerular filtration rate, probably as a result of renal vasoconstriction and it is possible that this could account for the oliguria which precedes migraine, and the increased urinary excretion of histidine and lysine which has been reported in migraine.[105]

Recently, Sicuteri has sought to relate the periodic fluctuation in susceptibility to induced migraine to the monoamine oxidase (MOA) activity of blood platelets which reaches its lowest level the day after a migraine headache. This supports the finding of Sandler et al[162] that MAO levels are low at the time of a migraine attack.

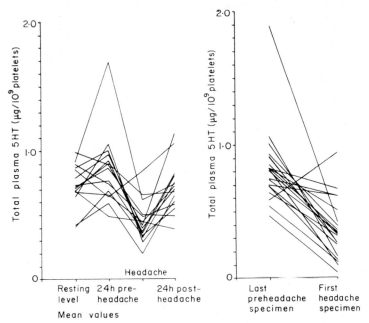

Figure 10.4. The mean values for plasma serotonin before, during and after migraine headache. The increased level of serotonin before the headache starts does not reach statistical significance but the fall during the attack is highly significant (P = <0.001). The graph on the right shows individual values before and after the onset of headache. (Adapted from Lance, Anthony and Hinterberger, 1967.) (Reproduced by courtesy of the editors of 'Archives of Neurology')

Prostaglandins

The prostaglandins are a group of lipid-soluble, unsaturated hydroxy acids which were named because of their presence in semen, which is responsible for the stimulation of uterine contraction on contact. They have since been found in many other body tissues. All the prostaglandins contain 20 carbon atoms and are fatty acids with the same carbon skeleton 'prostanoic acid', containing a cyclopentane ring, but have been classified according to the presence or absence of hydroxy and keto groups and the number of double bonds in the ring structure. The degree of unsaturation of the side-chains is indicated by the numeral after the classifying letter. The PGE series are vasodepressor agents and decrease uterine motility whereas the PGF series have the opposite effect. Both groups tend to increase gastrointestinal contraction. The PGA series have similar effects to the PGEs on the vascular system but have no gastro-intestinal activity[19b].

Interest in the possible relationship of prostaglandins to migraine was aroused by the observation of Carlson, Ekelund and Orö[36] that the intravenous infusion of PGE_1 into 8 healthy male subjects induced flushing (followed by pallor with higher doses), abdominal cramps, nausea and headache which became severe. In one patient the headache was unilateral and was preceded by the sensation of flashes of light. The authors quote an earlier experiment in which one of three normal subjects experienced visual symptoms in the form of 'lightnings and other coloured phenomena' with headache while PGE_1 was being infused. Neither subject had previously suffered from migraine. Arterial levels of free fatty acids in blood plasma increased in all subjects. The authors commented that the infusion of serotonin in man induces a similar flushing as well as a rise in free fatty acid concentration. They also remark that PGE_1 may disrupt mast cells and release heparin. They noted a marked decrease in systemic resistance which would be consistent with the opening of arterio-venous shunts. These observations invite comparison with those of Heyck[90] on the decreased arteriovenous oxygen difference in blood perfusing the scalp in the migraine attack, those of Hockaday et al[93] on the elevation of free fatty acids in the blood at this time, and those on degranulation of mast and basophil cells during migraine headache.[168,193,194]

There is evidence for a circulating oxytocic lipid during menstruation, and the presence of prostaglandins in the menstrual fluid suggests that these substances may play a part in the induction of menstruation.[94b] If this be the case, the liberation of prostaglandins by the hormonal changes at the end of the menstrual cycle could play a part in the course of menstrual migraine.

Sandler[162a] has sought to detect prostaglandins in venous blood and cerebrospinal fluid during the migraine attack without success but has pointed out that prostaglandins are largely removed on passage of blood through the lungs. He comments that serotonin and tyratamine have been shown to release prostaglandins from the lung in animal experiments, and advances the ingenious hypothesis that changes in serotonin or other triggering agents may release a prostaglandin or other vasoactive substance into the systemic circulation to act on receptors in the cranial vessels to produce the vascular changes of migraine. Sandler quotes a thesis by Alabaster which mentions that methysergide blocks the prostaglandin-liberating action of serotonin in the perfused lung.

It is possible that the prostaglandins may prove to be a link in the chain that binds the studies of serotonin, tyramine and oestrogens together in the genesis of migraine.

CONCLUSIONS

There is good evidence to consider migraine as an hereditary, paroxysmal vascular instability, each episode of which comprises a phase of arterial vasoconstriction, mainly intracranial, and a phase of arterial vasodilatation, mainly extracranial. One phase commonly follows the other, but the two may coexist so that focal neurological symptoms may appear when headache is established. Other forms of vascular headache caused by dilatation of the intracranial vessels may result from hypoxia, hypercapnia, hypoglycaemia, toxins or slowing of the circulation, but there is no evidence for these factors being operative in migraine except as an occasional trigger mechanism. The lumen of cerebral and scalp vessels may be altered reflexly during psychological conditioning,[214] but it is difficult to see how neural stimuli could be responsible for migraine when attacks have continued despite surgical assaults on every relevant nerve pathway. Furthermore, there is no physiological circumstance of which migraine might be considered an exaggerated or pathological form.

On the other hand, there is definite evidence of a disturbance in plasma serotonin in migraine and a suggestion that catecholamines might also be implicated. Migraine may thus prove to be a disorder of humoral vascular control. It has been shown that serotonin exerts a powerful constrictor effect on extracranial arteries in man when injected into the common carotid artery and it is reasonable to assume that it normally exerts some degree of tonic vasoconstrictor effect. The effect of serotonin on scalp capillaries has not been documented, but in view of the fact that patients complain of flushing of the face during intravenous injection of serotonin, it is probable that the usual effect is dilator, as it is on capillaries in most other areas of the body, and in other species. If this be so, sudden withdrawal of circulating serotonin would cause dilatation of scalp arteries with relative constriction of smaller vessels, thus increasing intra-arterial pressure with consequent distension of the arterial wall.

129

The fall of plasma serotonin at the onset of the migraine attack appears to be specific and not simply a reaction to headache, vomiting or stress. Migraine is precipitated when serotonin levels are lowered artificially by the injection of reserpine and is ameliorated by the injection of serotonin. These facts suggest that changes in serotonin levels are implicated in the mechanism of migraine and are not just an interesting association.

What causes the fall in plasma serotonin? The variable increase in urinary 5HIAA in the first 12 hours of some migraine attacks indicates that catabolism of serotonin may be increased at this time, which may be one factor. Platelets are known to take up serotonin as blood circulates through areas rich in serotonin, chiefly the gut. Atony of the gut associated with the anorexia and nausea of migraine could reduce the availability of serotonin supplies because it has been shown that plasma levels of serotonin vary with intestinal activity. In this event, the onset of vomiting and diarrhoea in migraine should help release serotonin from gut stores into the circulation, providing that the platelets are able to bind the serotonin. The latter is probably the main factor operating since plasma serotonin does not change substantially after the vomiting or diarrhoea of migraine.[7] It is interesting that many patients state that vomiting relieves their headache and that some try to induce vomiting for this reason.

The release of serotonin during blood clotting is associated with loss of ATP from platelets, but serotonin depletion in a spontaneous migraine headache occurs without ATP breakdown just as it does after injection of reserpine. It is therefore probable that some endogenous substance, with a reserpine-like action on platelets, is liberated at the onset of the migraine attack and that the consequent lowering of plasma serotonin initiates the vascular changes responsible for migraine headache.

Whatever the humoral changes which take place, certain scalp vessels must be hypersensitive in migraine since the pain is commonly unilateral, and the artificial lowering of serotonin levels by means of reserpine will induce a dull, bilateral headache in normal subjects, but not the paroxysms of migraine. It is also necessary to explain the intense pain of migraine which is not experienced with the physiological arterial dilatation of heat or exertion. There may be imbalance between the dilated arteries and constricted arterioles and capillaries, with consequent vascular overdistension and a sterile inflammatory response. Possibly serotonin is adsorbed to the arterial wall, sensitizing it to the action of bradykinin and other pain-causing agents.

130

SUMMARY

The mechanism of intracranial vasoconstriction remains obscure, but the increase in plasma serotonin, which is consistently observed before the start of the migraine attack, may later prove to be of relevance to the production of neurological symptoms as well as pre-headache oliguria and possibly mood changes. The investigation of serotonin uptake by cranial vessels and the action of prostaglandins may throw further light on the problem of intracranial vasoconstriction. Based on the foregoing fact and speculation, a possible mechanism for the migraine attack is illustrated in *Figure 10.5.*

SUMMARY

There is good evidence that the pain of migraine is caused by dilatation of cranial arteries, the greater component coming from the extracranial or scalp arteries. In addition to vascular distension and increased blood flow, there is a 'sterile inflammation' of the arterial wall, which may depend upon the local accumulation of pain-producing substances.

The focal neurological symptoms of migraine are probably initiated by intracranial vasoconstriction, but a secondary process of 'spreading depression' may account for the slowly progressive impairment of cortical function.

Neural control of cranial and extracranial blood vessels is mediated almost entirely by the sympathetic nervous system. There is no evidence of tonic vasoconstrictor action on these vessels except in the ear, which appears to have a different control mechanism from the scalp and forehead and cerebral vessels. Vasoconstriction may be induced experimentally by stimulation of the cervical sympathetic trunk, more so in extracranial than intracranial vessels, but it is doubtful whether this has physiological significance since vasoconstrictor reflexes are virtually absent from forehead and scalp. In contrast, vasodilator reflexes are active in these areas and depend upon sympathetic fibres travelling with cutaneous nerves. At present, there is no convincing evidence that the neural control of blood vessels is impaired in migraine, that migraine is caused by an abnormal neural discharge, or that operation on nerve pathways will interrupt the course of the migraine attack.

The possible role of prostaglandins in the genesis of migraine is at present under investigation.

Of the humoral agents which are known to have vasoactive properties, there is no evidence to implicate acetylcholine or histamine in the mechanism of migraine. Catabolites of norepinephrine and serotonin are excreted in the urine in excess in the early part of

131

POSSIBLE ROLE OF 5HT IN MIGRAINE

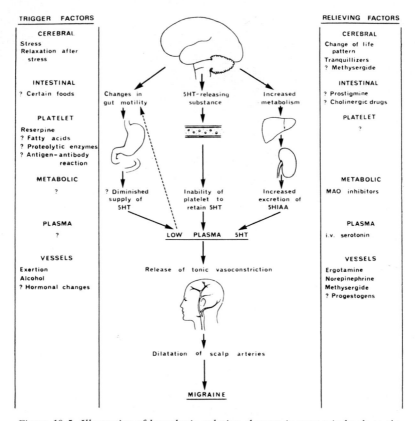

Figure 10.5. Illustration of hypothesis, relating changes in serotonin levels to the migraine attack. A serotonin-releasing factor has been demonstrated in the plasma during migraine headache, although its nature and origin are unknown. The consequent lowering of plasma serotonin withdraws vasoconstrictive support from extracranial vessels which then dilate to cause migraine headache. Possible trigger factors for migraine and the corresponding relieving factors are listed under the appropriate stages of the postulated mechanism. The brain is shown at the top of the diagram in deference to the author's neurological background without any firm conviction that it is the primary seat of disorder. (Reproduced by courtesy of the editors of 'Headache')

the migraine attack and plasma serotonin drops sharply at the onset of migraine, but not in other forms of headache. Since serotonin constricts scalp arteries in man, a fall in plasma serotonin may play a part in the extracranial vasodilatation characteristic of migraine (Figure 10.5). Serotonin changes are caused by the presence of a serotonin-releasing factor in the plasma during migraine headache and not due to any alteration in the serotonin-binding capacity of platelets. The reason why migraine is commonly unilateral is uncertain, but can be ascribed to an hereditary vascular instability, with hypersensitivity of the cranial blood vessels to humoral agents.

11—The Treatment of Migraine

Willis in 1684 wrote of migraine in a noble lady and stated that 'this Distemper . . . having pitched its tents near the confines of the Brain, had so long besieged its regal tower, yet it had not taken it . . . . There was no kind of Medicines both Cephalicks, Antiscorbuticks, Hysterical, all famous Specificks, which she took not, both from the Learned and the unlearned, from Quacks, and old Women, and yet notwithstanding she professed, that she had received from no Remedy, or method of Curing, any thing of Cure or Ease, but that the Contumacious and rebellious Disease, refused to be tamed, being deaf to the charms of every Medicine.[124]

Much is known about migraine and much can be done for the patient who is subject to it, but there is no complete and satisfying 'cure'. Migraine does not destroy life but can destroy the joy, value and rewards of living. It is a disease which warrants full attention from the general practitioner, who should be the person most qualified to treat it. Treatment starts with a consideration of the patient as well as his disease.

Personality and Problems

While the history and physical examination is in progress, there is time for some degree of mutual understanding to be established between doctor and patient, even if the two have never met before. Sometimes patients will discuss embarrassing personal problems more freely with an outsider than they would with a doctor who knows them and their family socially. Such a discussion takes time and tolerance, and may not be productive in finding solutions for the problems which emerge. However, it gives patients a chance to unburden themselves, the opportunity to obtain objective advice, and often reassurance that their problem is not unique and has been overcome by many others. A manipulation of the patient's personality or life pattern is not usually possible but the very fact of free discussion helps the patient and gives confidence that the doctor understands he is dealing with an individual.

134

Many migrainous patients exhibit the same qualities of anxiety and depression which characterize the sufferer from tension headache and must be treated accordingly. Relaxation exercises, and the judicious use of tranquillizers or antidepressant drugs thus have a place in the management of migraine as well as muscle-contraction headache. It must be emphasized that these measures are rarely sufficient to prevent migraine although they may reduce the frequency of attacks. The author has known a handful of patients who are completely free of headaches while they are on vacation or enjoying a pleasant overseas trip or a cruise at sea, but has also known many more who have experienced disappointment that whatever they do or wherever they go, their headaches pursue them, even to the Great Barrier Reef or the tranquil shores of Tahiti.

Diet

During the history-taking, certain foods may have been mentioned which are said to precipitate migraine headache. Many of these will trigger a headache only when a patient is in a susceptible phase. The author knows of some who can drink red wines with impunity for some days after a spontaneous migraine attack, but avoid them after this 'refractory period', as a glass of claret will then bring on an attack. There is undoubtedly a big element of psychological conditioning in this, but it is sensible for patients to avoid any article of diet which they think might be responsible for their attacks. There is certainly no reason for giving general advice to all migrainous patients to avoid fatty foods, chocolates or oranges, because trigger factors are very much an individual affair. Dr. A. G. Child kindly skin-tested 34 of our migrainous patients for food and other allergies. Twenty-three patients who gave positive reactions avoided the appropriate allergens for several months under supervision, without reduction in the frequency of attacks. Ten patients were placed on low-fat diets under the direction of Dr. Joan Woodhill, for up to 6 months, but again the pattern of attacks remained unaltered. It is thus unlikely that any change in diet will make a substantial difference to the migraine patient.

The oral administration of the bacterium *Lactobacillus acidophilus* has been claimed to improve 8 out of the 10 patients with migraine in whom it was used by altering the intestinal flora and presumably having some effect on intestinal absorption. The author has not used this treatment in a sufficient number of patients to be able to comment on its efficacy except to say that the degree of improvement in a handful of patients has not been remarkable. The prevention of hypoglycaemia by taking regular meals and a late supper before retiring may be desirable for other reasons but does not prevent migraine. Stimulation of gastrointestinal motility by neostigmine and similar drugs has been employed in the past. The release of serotonin from gut stores by neostigmine provides a possible reason for its use, but the author has had no experience with it.

Exercise

Standing on the head improves vasoconstrictor reflexes in scalp arteries[214] and has a rational basis for the gymnastically adroit, but is of limited application.

Hormones

Hormonal factors are of importance in migraine and the use of progestogenic agents and injections of chorionic gonadotrophin have been recommended in treatment. In 1962, Lundberg[128] reported that 55 of 84 patients (including 6 men) became free of migraine attacks when treated with methylnortestosterone 1–2 mg daily or allyloestrenol 2·5–15 mg daily, given for three weeks of the menstrual cycle, or continuously. Continuous administration caused amenorrhoea in most cases. Menstrual disturbances occurred in 36 out of 76 women with cyclical therapy and 9 noticed hirsutes, acne or hoarseness. We followed up this report by using allyloestrenol in the dosage recommended in a pilot trial of 20 patients. The results were disappointing and did not warrant the organization of a controlled trial. Recently a new progestogenic agent, flumedroxone, the use of which had also been advocated by Lundberg, was subjected to a controlled trial in which its effect was compared with that of methysergide over a period of 9 months in 35 patients.[95] There was no significant difference between the number of attacks per month experienced before the trial period and the number of monthly attacks while taking flumedroxone. This contrasted with the improvement of all but 3 patients taking methysergide.

Gonadotrophic hormone has been used in the treatment of migraine for more than 30 years.[155a] We have given gonadotrophic hormone 500 I.U. twice weekly to 26 patients for periods of 2–10 months. Only 10 showed worthwhile improvement and it was felt that this result, which may well have been due to the natural history of the disease, did not warrant the trouble and expense of regular injections.

Various forms of contraceptive pill make migraine worse in most instances, and permanent neurological deficit has been reported in 6 patients whose vasoconstrictive phase of migraine was prolonged while taking oral contraceptives.[78]

The only hormonal treatment which is at least 60 per cent effective is pregnancy.

Prevention of Salt and Water Retention

Fluid retention is common for several days before the menstrual period and is also common immediately before migraine headache. The fact that menstruation and migraine often coincide led to the use of salt restriction and diuretics in the treatment of migraine whether or not it tended to occur with the menses. Fluid retention may indeed be prevented by such measures but migraine usually continues unabated.[163]

Histamine Desensitization

Histamine, given by incrementing subcutaneous injections or weekly intravenous infusions, has been used in the treatment of migraine for many years. This is a difficult procedure to adapt to a controlled trial to see whether it really is effective. A follow-up for 8 months after a course of three intravenous infusions at weekly intervals revealed that 21 per cent of patients became headache-free and another 42 per cent were more than half-improved.[166] It is not known whether this treatment has some non-specific effect on vascular reactivity, or whether its action is purely psychological.

Manipulative and Surgical Procedures

Success has been claimed for manipulation of the neck in the treatment of migraine headache as in many other fields, but objective evidence is lacking. Cyriax[51] stated that 'an attack of migraine can sometimes be instantly aborted by strong traction on the neck. Half a minute's traction in some cases is regularly successful, in others not. The mechanism is obscure (it may be connected with the stretching of the carotid artery) and the phenomenon would clearly repay further study . . .'. Cyriax goes on to say 'A minority of patients have reported to me, some years after the reduction by manipulation of a cervical disc, that since that time attacks of obvious migraine have ceased'. Such improvement has only been noted in middle-aged patients, not in the young, and Cyriax postulates that pressure by osteophytes on the vertebral artery and the nerve plexus surrounding it may therefore play some part in the production of migraine. Since many patients have already undergone cervical manipulation without success by the time they are referred to a neurologist, the author remains sceptical, although prepared to

THE TREATMENT OF MIGRAINE

alter his views should any controlled observations be published. The author wonders whether manipulating the neck is really a sophisticated way of pulling the patient's leg.

Surgical procedures were discussed in the previous chapter and it was concluded that operations on sympathetic or parasympathetic nerve pathways, and ligation of branches of the external carotid or middle meningeal arteries or both did not provide any lasting benefit.

Pharmacotherapy

At present, the unpalatable fact has to be accepted that psychological readjustment, physiological measures and manipulative or surgical procedures do little to alter the natural history of migraine. The management of migraine still depends on pharmacotherapy.

The drug treatment of migraine falls into the following categories:

(1) Drugs which constrict the extracranial arteries such as ergotamine tartrate, dihydroergotamine, and 1-methylergotamine hydrogen tartrate (MY25). Serotonin and noradrenaline have also been used experimentally for this purpose.

(2) Serotonin antagonists, some of which simulate the action of serotonin in potentiating the effect of vasoconstrictor agents: methysergide (Deseril, Sansert), cyproheptadine (Periactin), pizotifen (BC105, Sandomigran), methylergol carbamide maleate (Lysenyl).

(3) Drugs blocking beta adrenergic receptors on blood vessels, thereby diminishing vasodilator responses, e.g. propranalol (Inderal) and prindolol (LB46, Visken).

(4) Drugs which block central vasomotor reflexes and diminish vascular reactivity such as clonidine (Catapres).

(5) Monoamine oxidase inhibitors, such as phenelzine (Nardil), which permit the accumulation of serotonin and other vasoactive amines such as noradrenaline.

(6) A miscellaneous group comprising anticonvulsants, such as carbamazepine (Tegretol); Levodopa; indomethacin (Indocid, Indocin); and methdilazine (Tacaryl, Dilosyn), which has anti-bradykinin properties.

THE MECHANISM OF ACTION OF PHARMACEUTICAL AGENTS

Ergot derivatives and serotonin antagonists

It is generally believed that ergotamine tartrate is effective in relieving migraine by constricting scalp arteries. Unfortunately it frequently induces nausea and vomiting, so that it would be desirable to synthesize a related preparation in which the vasoconstrictive property was separated from the emetic side-effects. Berde and his colleagues[19] have shown that the vasoconstrictor activity of ergotamine compounds depends upon the pre-existing vascular resistance. Working with the perfused dog hind-limb they found that ergotamine, dihydroergotamine (DHE) and 1-methylergotamine (MY25) act as vasoconstrictors when the vascular resistance is low but are transformed into vasodilators as the vascular resistance is increased. The strength and long duration of the antiserotonin effect of ergotamine and 1-methylergotamine are similar but the vasoconstrictive property of ergotamine is 5–100 times that of 1-methylergotamine when tested in different preparations. Indeed 1-methylergotamine will actually inhibit the induction of gangrene in the rat's tail by ergotamine. The oxytocic effect of 1-methylergotamine is approximately 1 per cent of that of ergotamine and it has no emetic effect in the dog.

It is probable that ergotamine derivatives prevent the re-uptake of noradrenaline into body stores thereby increasing the amount of noradrenaline available for adherence to the alpha adrenergic receptors which are responsible for constrictor effects. Berde (personal communication) has recently emphasized the possible significance of capacitance vessels in the microcirculation, the part of the venous compartment which follows the postcapillary resistance vessels. Low frequency sympathetic nerve stimulation increases the tone of the capacitance vessels and higher frequencies also contract the resistance vessels, particularly the precapillary resistance vessels. Ergotamine and dihydroergotamine have no effect on the precapillary sphincters but constrict the capacitance vessels, which decrease the blood content of the area and increase venous return. Hydergine (dihydroergocristine, dihydroergocornine and dihydroergokryptine) also dilates the precapillary sphincters. The part played by the capacitance vessels in migraine is as yet unknown but there is some evidence that they may be overdistended because of the facial and scalp oedema which has been reported on occasions, and that flow in this system may be slowed down because of blood being shunted away from the periphery.

The antiserotonin effect of methysergide is much greater than that of ergotamine and 1-methylergotamine in preventing serotonin-induced oedema of the rat's paw but its action is short-lived. If the agents are given more than 2 hours before the injection of serotonin, methysergide is less effective than the other two ergot derivatives.

139

The application of methysergide solution to the conjunctiva, or the oral administration of methysergide, does not directly constrict the conjunctival vessels but increases their sensitivity to the constrictor effects of noradrenaline.[53] Serotonin and methysergide were shown to have a similar effect in potentiating the vasoconstrictor effect of noradrenaline in the isolated perfused central artery of the rabbit ear by De la Lande, Cannell and Waterson.[57] Methysergide may thus act as a competitive antagonist to serotonin in man, an effect which has been demonstrated in the pulmonary circulation of sheep.[84] Serotonin or its precursor, 5 hydroxytryptophan, inhibits various pressor and depressor reflexes in animals, and methysergide has a similar, although weaker effect in man.[52,53] The beneficial effect of methysergide may lie in simulating the action of serotonin in helping to preserve tonic vasoconstriction of scalp arteries when the plasma serotonin level drops during the migraine attack.

More recently, Carroll and Glover[38] have studied the effects of caffeine, dihydroergotamine, 1-methylergotamine (MY25) pizotifen (BC105, Sandomigran), cyproheptadine and methysergide on the rabbit's ear artery preparation and have observed the way in which these agents alter the arterial response to serotonin, noradrenaline and histamine.

Dihydroergotamine and MY25 were found to constrict the artery for periods in excess of 2 hours, although the dose of MY25 required was some 50 times greater than that of DHE. Methysergide produced a brief contraction, as did caffeine when used in very high dosage. Pizotifen and cyproheptadine had no discernible effect in any dose. The response of the artery to methysergide was comparable to the constriction produced by serotonin and gave a parallel log-dose response, thus supporting the hypothesis that it may occupy the same arterial receptor sites as serotonin. The prior administration of pizotifen or cyproheptadine blocked the arterial response to serotonin and methysergide, but not the response to noradrenaline, DHE or MY25. When each of the substances under test was injected before an injection of serotonin, all were found to antagonize the effect of serotonin, the most potent being pizotifen and cyproheptadine which blocked the serotonin effect for more than 2 hours. Methysergide was only one third to one sixth as potent and its serotonin antagonism lasted for only 5–10 minutes.

Serotonin potentiated the constriction produced by noradrenaline in the rabbit ear artery and the same effect was noted with DHE, methysergide and MY25 although their potency with respect to serotonin was only half to a quarter, one tenth to one twenty-fifth and one fiftieth to a two hundredth respectively. These substances also potentiated the vasoconstrictor effect of serotonin itself although an injection of serotonin did not potentiate subsequent injections of serotonin. Pizotifen and cyproheptadine demonstrated noradrenaline antagonism and did not potentiate vasoconstriction at any dose level. Pizotifen was capable of blocking the direct vasoconstrictor effect of serotonin while leaving the potentiation of noradrenaline by serotonin unchanged.

Histamine constricted the rabbit ear artery and both pizotifen and cyproheptadine proved very effective in blocking this response. On the other hand, DHE, methysergide and MY25 all potentiated the histamine response in low doses, although it was blocked by larger doses.

It can be seen therefore that pizotifen and cyproheptadine are the most effective antagonists of both serotonin and histamine in this experimental arrangement. If the migraine attack depended upon the adsorption of serotonin to the vessel wall, one would expect these two agents to be the most useful in the relief of migraine. If, on the other hand, the relief of migraine depends upon the potentiation of arterial vasoconstriction by noradrenaline in the absence of the naturally occurring serotonin, then methysergide should prove more effective. The dominant action of DHE and MY25 appears to be one of direct constriction of arteries and not to be secondary to that of the vasoactive amines.

Beta Adrenergic Blocking Agents

The dilatation of peripheral arteries in response to adrenaline is thought to be due to the uptake of adrenaline by beta receptors in the vessel wall. Beta blockade could therefore prevent dilatation in response to any humoral agent employing these receptors. There have been isolated reports of the effectiveness of propranolol (Inderal) in reducing the frequency and severity of migraine, including one double-blind trial in which 15 of 19 patients improved.[206] A new beta blocker, pindolol (or prinodolol) (Visken) has an indole ring structure although its side-chain is typical of this group of drugs. Pindolol proved to be 10–40 times more potent than propranolol as a beta adrenergic blocking agent in animal experiments and in human volunteers, and has given promising results in our own comparative trials,[12] but two double-blind trials in Scandinavia[62b,176c] have recently given negative results. Further trials are required before firm recommendations can be made about this group of drugs.

141

Clonidine

A new hypotensive agent, 2-(2,6-dichlorophenylamino) 2-imidazoline hydrochloride, known as clonidine (Catapres, Dixarit) has been reported as being a useful prophylactic agent for migraine,[213,217] Sjaastad and Stensrud[176b] recently submitted 26 migrainous patients to a double-blind trial in which 16 patients experienced less headache while taking clonidine 75 μg daily than placebo. Clonidine is not a ganglion-blocking agent, is without effect on alpha and beta adrenergic receptors and does not deplete tissues of their catecholamine content. Zaimis and Hanington[217] found that pretreatment with clonidine reduced the vasoconstrictor response of the cat femoral artery to noradrenaline, adrenaline and angiotensin as well as diminishing the vasodilator effect of isoprenaline, so that it damps down both constrictor and dilator responses. Cineangiographic studies in man have shown that the intravenous injection of clonidine 75 μg speeds up the cerebral circulation time.

Monamine Oxidase Inhibitors

Since serotonin levels are lowered in migraine, the use of a drug which maintains or increases serotonin levels is a logical form of treatment and a number of favourable reports concerning MAO inhibitors have appeared in the past.[27] Anthony and Lance[10] treated 25, patients who had failed to respond to other forms of interval medication, with phenelzine 45 mg daily for periods up to 2 years. The frequency of headache was reduced to less than half in 20 of the 25 patients. Although mean plasma serotonin increased by about 50 per cent there was no correlation between the serotonin level and response of each individual patient.

Indomethacin (Indocid, Indocin)

When used in a large dose (150–200 mg daily) indomethacin is said to be beneficial in preventing migraine.[172] Large doses produce a high incidence of gastrointestinal side-effects and may possibly be dangerous. A controlled trial of indomethacin, using the conventional dosage of 25 mg three times daily, showed that the drug was no more effective than placebo.[9]

Anticonvulsants

Carbamazepine (Tegretol) is now accepted as an anticonvulsant and an agent for the control of trigeminal neuralgia. In a recent

142

double-blind cross-over trial, 45 patients experienced a total of 30 migraine attacks in six weeks while taking carbamazepine and 48 patients suffered 186 attacks while on placebo for six weeks.[158] Of patients treated with carbamazepine, 84 per cent improved while only 27 per cent of patients improved while taking placebo medication. The number of patients who improved markedly or achieved complete control was 26 (57·7 per cent). Side-effects such as giddiness, drowsiness and nausea were noticed by two-thirds of patients but were sufficient to discontinue treatment in only 1 of 45 patients. These results were not confirmed in a recent comparative trial from our clinic[12] and we found that 12 of 51 patients had to cease treatment because of side-effects.

Bradykinin Antagonist

Methdilazine (Tacaryl, Dilosyn) is an N-substituted phenothiazine derivative with strong antihistamine and antibradykinin activity, and weak antiserotonin effects. When used as prophylactic therapy for migraine in the dose of 8–16 mg morning and night it improved 41 per cent of patients which was not significantly better than the placebo rate of 31 per cent.[119] Drowsiness was a common side-effect.

Levodopa

The use of L-dopa for Parkinson's disease has been said to benefit migraine in those patients who suffer from both disorders, but there is still doubt about this.

TREATMENT OF THE ACUTE ATTACK OF MIGRAINE

Since the present concept of migraine headache is one of painful dilatation of cranial vessels, the object of handling an acute attack is to induce constriction of the scalp arteries, and to relieve pain and vomiting. Intravenous injection of serotonin or infusion of noradrenaline have been used experimentally to induce vasoconstriction with success in terminating migraine headache. These measures cause unpleasant side-effects and are not practicable for routine use. The agent accepted as safe and effective for some 40 years is ergotamine tartrate, which is considered to relieve the pain of migraine headache in about 70 per cent of patients. In one analysis of the response of 263 patients to treatment, ergotamine-containing preparations regularly relieved the headaches completely in 47 per cent and partially in 34 per cent.[166] It is common for patients to state that their headaches last only 2–3 hours if they have access to ergotamine tartrate and for 12–24 hours if they do not. Some patients who vomit early in their attack are not helped by oral ergotamine tartrate but obtain rapid relief from the use of suppositories. In view of this clinical experience, the report of Waters[203] that ergotamine tartrate 2–3 mg orally was no more effective in relieving migraine headache than placebo tablets was quite startling. Waters based his analysis on 79 women who had taken tablets for at least one headache in each 8 week treatment period. Of the original 129 women identified by questionnaire as having headaches which were probably migrainous in type, 50 were excluded either before or during the trial, 5 because they were already taking effective tablets, the nature of which was undisclosed. It is not clear whether those retained in the trial had previously been treated by some ergotamine preparation without success, whether they did indeed take their tablets early in the attack as instructed and whether they were subject to vomiting with their headache. The patients were followed up and assessed by a nurse. In a separate investigation 43 of the 79 women who completed the trial were examined by a neurologist who diagnosed 31 as having migraine. Sufficient doubt has been aroused by this trial to warrant a further investigation in which the clinical control is as stringent as the statistical control.

In the meantime it seems justifiable to reiterate the time-honoured advice that ergotamine tartrate should be given at the first indication of a migraine attack, in adequate dosage (1–4 mg depending on the patient's weight and tolerance), in a form which is readily absorbed and acceptable to the patient. Nausea is a common side-effect and some patients complain of aching muscles. Vasoconstrictive phenomena are uncommon with the usual therapeutic doses of ergotamine tartrate but the appearance of signs of peripheral ischaemia may prevent its further use. Ergotamine tartrate has a slight oxytocic effect and should be used with caution in pregnancy. Habituation to ergot preparations may lead a migrainous patient to take daily medication, with a rebound headache developing every time the tablets are omitted. Supervised withdrawal in hospital may then become necessary.

There are now many preparations available, thus giving patients scope for experimentation to see which suits them best.

Ergotamine Tartrate

(a) Coated tablets of ergotamine tartrate 1 mg (Femergin, Gynergen). 1–3 tablets should be swallowed at the onset of a migraine attack and repeated in half an hour if necessary. One tablet is usually sufficient as an initial dose for a child and two for most adults. If the attack is not aborted by the suggested two doses at half-hourly intervals, there is no point in taking more.

(b) Uncoated tablets of ergotamine tartrate 1 mg (Ergomar, Lingraine). These should be dissolved in the mouth and are then absorbed supposedly from the buccal mucosa. They were considered to act more rapidly than coated tablets by 40 per cent of our patients but some objected to their taste. The dosage schedule is the same for coated tablets.

(c) Aerosol form (Medihaler). A fine powder of ergotamine tartrate is available in a pressure pack for inhalation. Instructions must be followed carefully so that the powder is inhaled deeply into the lungs. The device delivers 0·36 mg ergotamine at a time, and the inhalation can be repeated up to 6 times at intervals of 5 minutes.

(d) Injection. Ergotamine tartrate may be given by subcutaneous or intramuscular injection in doses of 0·25–0·5 mg.

Compounds Containing Ergotamine Tartrate

Cafergot.—Ergotamine tartrate 1 mg is combined with caffeine 100 mg in Cafergot tablets which are swallowed, or Cafergot-Q tablets which may be chewed for more rapid absorption.

Cafergot-PB suppositories.—Suppositories containing ergotamine tartrate 2 mg, caffeine 100 mg, belladonna alkaloids 0·25 mg and isobutyl allyl barbituric acid 100 mg. One suppository is inserted rectally at the onset of migraine and this may be repeated in one hour if necessary. This form is particularly useful for those patients who become nauseated early in the attack when gastric absorption is impaired. Cramps in the thighs and drowsiness are not uncommon as side-effects.

Migral, Migril—These tablets contain ergotamine tartrate 2 mg, caffeine 100 mg, with cyclizine 50 mg as an antiemetic. One tablet is taken at the onset of migraine and repeated in half an hour if necessary.

Ergodryl—Ergotamine tartrate 1 mg, caffeine 100 mg, with diphenhydramine 25 mg as an antiemetic. One or two capsules are taken at the onset and repeated in half an hour if necessary.

There are a number of other combinations, containing different antiemetics, belladonna alkaloids or analgesics.

Indomethacin (Indocid, Indocin)

It has been reported that the intravenous administration of indomethacin will prevent the development of migraine in most patients[172] but the author is not personally familiar with its use in this manner.

Drugs to Relieve Pain and Vomiting

Once a severe migraine headache is established, ergotamine tartrate is rarely of use and there is no alternative to symptomatic treatment with analgesics. The intravenous or intramuscular injection of diazepam (Valium) 10 mg may be helpful as an antiemetic agent or one of the phenothiazine group such as prochlorperazine (Stemetil) 12·5 mg or thiethylperazine dimaleate (Torecan) 10 mg may be required to suppress vomiting. The latter group may occasionally give rise to dystonic reactions, so that it is worth having an ampoule of benztropine mesylate (Cogentin) 2 mg available for intravenous injection should this occur.

PREVENTION OF FREQUENT ATTACKS BY INTERVAL MEDICATION

The prevention of migraine headache by continuous medication is a comparatively recent advance in the treatment of this disorder. When the frequency of migraine increases to two or more attacks each month, interval therapy must be considered. Before regular medication is started, it is important to consider whether one of the following factors could be responsible for the stepping up in intensity of the migrainous onslaught.

(1) Increased emotional or mental stress, such as a trap situation in the patient's private life or work.

(2) The onset of a depressive state.

(3) Increase in systemic blood pressure.

(4) The use of the contraceptive pill.

(5) Too frequent use of preparations containing ergotamine.

If the frequency of migraine attacks persists after attention to any of these factors which are relevant, it usually becomes necessary to prescribe a prophylactic drug to be taken two or three times daily in an endeavour to prevent the headaches completely or at least ameliorate their severity.

Sedatives and Antidepressant Drugs

Regular sedation is worth a trial in excitable children but is rarely effective in adults. Tranquillizing agents, such as diazepam (Valium) 2–5 mg or chlordiazepoxide (Librium) 10 mg three times daily are useful in those patients in whom nervous tension is playing a part in increasing the frequency of migraine attacks. Antidepressants, such as amitriptyline (Tryptanol, Tryptizol, Elavil, Laroxyl) 10–25 mg, or imipramine (Tofranil) 10–25 mg three times daily may be of considerable indirect benefit. It is probable that anticonvulsant and

146

antihistamine drugs have no advantage over other sedatives in the treatment of migraine. It must be remembered that fluctuations occur in the natural history of migraine, and the psychological boost of any new treatment will give a certain placebo response, amounting to 20–30 per cent of patients improved.[48,122]

Ergotamine Tartrate and Related Preparations

The use of ergotamine tartrate for prophylaxis is limited by the relatively short duration of its vasoconstrictor action, but some patients find that they can prevent a nocturnal or early morning attack of migraine by taking 1–2 mg on retiring. Barrie, Fox, Weatherall and Wilkinson[16] undertook a controlled trial of ergotamine tartrate 0·5 or 1·0 mg daily, ergometrine maleate 1·0 or 2·0 mg daily and methysergide maleate (Deseril, Sansert) 3·0 or 6·0 mg daily in 105 outpatients with frequent migraine attacks. They concluded that methysergide was marginally more effective than the other drugs but produced more side-effects.

A preparation containing phenobarbitone 20 mg, ergotamine tartrate 0·3 mg and belladonna alkaloids 0·1 mg (Bellergal), when given as one tablet three times daily, is more effective than simple sedation and gives improvement in about 35 per cent of patients.[48] This is a useful medication for children, one tablet each night often being sufficient to reduce substantially the frequency of migraine headache.

Dihydroergotamine (DHE) has been used for many years as a prophylactic agent for migraine, particularly in Europe, but the author is not aware of any comparative assessment of its merits. 1-methyl-ergotamine (MY25), which exerts a prolonged tonic vasoconstrictor effect similar to but milder than that of DHE, is at present being evaluated.

Serotonin Antagonists

These agents fall into two groups. The first, consisting of pizotifen (BC105, Sandomigran) and cyproheptadine (Periactin) do not directly constrict the vessel wall, have a potent antihistamine and antiserotonin action and show no evidence of potentiating the vasoconstrictor action of serotonin or noradrenaline.

The second group, consisting of methysergide (Deseril, Sansert), DHE and MY25, exert some direct effects on the vessel wall, demonstrate relatively transient antiserotonin action but simulate serotonin in potentiating the constrictor response to noradrenaline.

Pizotifen (BC105, Sandomigran)

This is a benzo-cycloheptathiophene derivative with a basic side-chain resembling that of cyproheptadine. Sicuteri, Franchi and Del Bianco[171] reported that 70 per cent of patients with 3 or more migraine attacks each month were improved by therapy with pizotifen, and Sjaastad and Stensrud confirmed its effectiveness in a double-blind trial.[176a] An initial controlled trial in our clinic[114] was disappointing in that only 12 out of 25 patients responded, but in an extended trial 31 out of 53 patients who were given pizotifen as an initial treatment improved substantially and the improvement rate in a total of 103 patients was 50 per cent.[119] Drowsiness, increase in appetite, and gain in weight were common side-effects. Pizotifen is prescribed as 0·5 mg tablets, the daily dose varying between 1·0 and 3·0 mg.

Cyproheptadine (Periactin)

In two comparative trials[48,119] we have found the improvement rates with methysergide, cyproheptadine and placebo to be 64, 46 and 20 per cent and 64, 43 and 32 per cent respectively. Cyproheptadine is prescribed as 4 mg tablets, the daily dose varying between 8 and 32 mg daily. The side-effects are similar to those of pizotifen, drowsiness being the most common, with stimulation of appetite and weight gain being important secondary symptoms.

Methysergide (Deseril, Sansert)

Methysergide has proven the most useful prophylactic agent in migraine.[47] Regular medication with methysergide 2–6 mg daily suppresses migraine completely in about 26 per cent of patients and improves substantially another 40 per cent.[48] About 40 per cent of patients experience side-effects, chiefly abdominal discomfort and muscle cramps, when treatment is first started but these usually pass off after some days or weeks. Less common side-effects include insomnia, depression, a sensation of swelling in the face or throat, increase in the venules over the nose and cheeks, and gain in weight.[47,48] Any medication which prevents migraine may lead to gain in weight, because 'eating days' are substituted for 'vomiting days'. About 10 per cent of patients are unable to tolerate methysergide because of persistent unpleasant symptoms or the appearance of peripheral vasoconstriction with pallor of the extremities, intermittent claudication, or, very rarely, angina pectoris. These symptoms disappear on ceasing medication or, if mild, may be overcome by combining a vasodilator drug with methysergide.[122]

Case Report

A woman aged 59 years had suffered approximately eight attacks of right hemicrania monthly for the past 5 years. After 1 month on methysergide, 6 mg daily, she was free of headache but complained of weakness and numbness of her left hand. Examination revealed that the left radial pulse was absent and the small muscles of the left hand were weak. Methysergide was suspended and a vasodilator agent* substituted. Power returned within 2 days and the left radial pulse was palpable when she was examined 1 week later. The patient then experienced second daily right hemicrania for 1 month. Methysergide and the vasodilator drug in combination restored the patient's freedom from headache without further weakness or numbness of her left hand.

Peripheral vascular disease, coronary artery disease, hypertension, a history of thrombophlebitis or peptic ulcer, and pregnancy, are all relative, but not absolute, contra-indications to the use of methysergide.[47] The reason for avoiding methysergide in the first four conditions is fairly clear, since arterial vasoconstriction is a recognized side-effect. The administration of methysergide was found to double basal gastric secretion of hydrochloric acid in 6 patients with peptic ulcer, and hence its use is best avoided in this condition. There is no evidence to suggest that methysergide is harmful to mother or foetus, but it has been our own practice to suspend its use once a patient becomes pregnant because of innate conservatism. Three of our patients continued with methysergide throughout pregnancy and bore normal full-term infants.

Retroperitoneal fibrosis, pleural fibrosis and cardiac valvular fibrosis developed in about 100 patients of the half-million who were estimated to have been treated with methysergide.[80] With the dosage recommended above, we have seen 1 patient with chronic pleural fibrosis and 1 with retroperitoneal fibrosis among more than 1,000 patients treated for up to 9 years. The symptoms of these fibrotic syndromes commonly resolve if methysergide treatment is ceased, but there is 1 reported instance of retroperitoneal fibrosis developing over a period of 6 months after methysergide was withdrawn.[165] It has been recommended that patients cease treatment for 1 month in every 6 to permit resolution of any impending fibrosis and no new cases have been reported since this became standard practice. Patients should see their physicians every few months while taking methysergide or report if they notice any unusual symptoms, since such fibrotic syndromes are uncommon and potentially reversible.

The fibrotic complications of methysergide may well be the result

---

* A proprietary combination of dihydroergocornine, dihydroergocristine and dihydroergokryptine (Hydergine).

of its serotonin-like action. Graham[80] has commented on the similarity of the appearance at operation of valvular fibrosis in methysergide-treated patients to that seen in carcinoid syndrome. The administration of serotonin to rats either decreases or increases granuloma formation, depending upon the function of the adrenal gland.[20] Excessive fibrosis appears only if adrenal insufficiency is induced. This raises the question of whether there might be adrenal insufficiency in patients who develop fibrotic syndromes in response to serotonin or methysergide. It is possible that any drug which relies upon a serotonin-simulating action for the treatment of migraine has the potential of producing excessive fibrosis in susceptible subjects.

Clonidine (*Dixarit, Catapres*) and Beta Adrenergic Blocking Agents

These substances are currently being evaluated and may well find a place in the interval therapy of migraine. We have found an improvement rate of 53 per cent with clonidine and 64 per cent with pindolol (Visken)[12]

Monoamine Oxidase Inhibitors

This form of treatment is of limited value because of potential hazards in the use of monoamine oxidase inhibitors which necessitate dietary restriction and the avoidance of other drugs. It should be reserved for those patients with severe migraine who are completely resistant to other forms of medication.

General Conclusions about the Drug Treatment of Migraine

When attacks are infrequent, it is pointless to prescribe interval medication. If the patient is able to anticipate when the next episode is coming because of the association with a precipitating factor, such as menstruation, or because of some sensation, such as an intense feeling of well-being, which regularly precedes an attack, then treatment may be planned accordingly. Ergotamine tartrate may be given the night before the migraine headache is anticipated, or methysergide may be started 24 hours before if there is sufficient warning.

The treatment of the acute attack still relies on an adequate dose of ergotamine tartrate given in the form most acceptable to the patient, usually as a tablet or suppository. The suppository is particularly useful in patients who vomit early in the headache and have no time to absorb oral medication.

In patients who are subject to two migraine headaches or more each month, a thorough trial of interval treatment should be given, much in the same way as anticonvulsants are used in epilepsy, with the object of eliminating the attacks completely. In children, it may be worth starting with simple sedation. In adults, sedation alone is rarely helpful and my own practice is to start with pizotifen 0·5 mg or cyproheptadine 4 mg two or three times daily for the first few days to ensure that the patient is not rendered unduly drowsy, then increase the dose up to two tablets three times daily, if necessary. If there has been no significant improvement at the end of a month the treatment is then changed to methysergide. Much has been written about the side-effects of methysergide but if used cautiously it is not hazardous, and it is certainly the most effective preparation at present available for the control of migraine.

It is advisable to give a trial dose of 1 mg and then to increase the dose at daily intervals from 1 mg twice daily up to 2 mg three times daily if necessary. The tablets are best taken after meals to minimize epigastric discomfort. Dosage and timing can be adjusted to suit the requirements of each particular patient. A patient who is invariably awakened at 3 a.m. by an attack may be controlled by nocturnal medication only. A woman whose attacks are more frequent with menstruation may require increased dosage at that time.

Patients who become virtually free of headache while taking 6 mg daily may slowly reduce the dose to the minimum which will maintain control. When a patient who has been maintained on methysergide ceases treatment for one month every six, it is advisable to withdraw the drug slowly in order to prevent a severe 'rebound headache'. Methysergide does not appear to have any curative effect and must be continued as long as the tendency to headache persists.

Methysergide is not effective for the treatment of the acute attack in most instances, although some patients whose frequency of headache has diminished under treatment may find that some episodes can be aborted by taking their dose of methysergide at the first symptom of an attack. Ergotamine preparations may be used for the acute attack in the usual way if some headaches occur while the patient is under treatment with methysergide, and are then often more effective than before.

Migraine is a difficult problem to treat but we can never say to a patient that his illness cannot be helped until we have tried conscientiously all kinds of medicines 'Cephalics, Hysterical, all famous Specificks'. Otherwise, as Willis foretold, our patients will turn to the unlearned, quacks and old women.

12—Cluster Headache (Migrainous Neuralgia)

Periodic migrainous neuralgia or cluster headache may be defined as a severe unilateral head or facial pain, which lasts for minutes or hours, associated commonly with ipsilateral lacrimation and blockage of the nostril, usually recurring once or more daily for a period of weeks or months. The term cluster headache derives from the tendency for the pain to appear in bouts, separated by intervals of complete freedom.[110]

In 1840, Romberg[157] described as 'ciliary neuralgia' recurrent pain in the eye, which was generally confined to one side and associated with photophobia. 'The pupil is contracted. The pain not infrequently extends over the head and face. The eye generally weeps and becomes red. These symptoms occur in paroxysms of a uniform or irregular character, and isolated or combined with facial neuralgia and hemicrania.' Romberg considered that scrofula was the main cause of ciliary neuralgia but that it was also brought on by discharges, especially seminal emissions. The condition was first recorded in the English medical literature by Harris in 1926 as ciliary (migrainous) neuralgia and this description was later elaborated.[86]

The uncertainty about the nature and aetiology of this disorder is reflected by other names which have been used to describe similar syndromes over the past century such as red migraine, erythroprosopalgia, erythromelalgia of the head, syndrome of hemicephalic vasodilation of sympathetic origin, autonomic faciocephalgia, greater superficial petrosal neuralgia and histamine cephalgia.[61,75,156,186] Symonds[189] used the non-committal title of 'a particular variety of headache'. Sphenopalatine neurosis[178] and vidian neuralgia[198] were described as affecting mostly female patients and appear more akin

152

to lower half headache, now known as facial migraine, than to the syndrome under discussion.

The nature of the attack and pattern of recurrence of this syndrome are so characteristic that it can readily be distinguished from migraine and trigeminal neuralgia. In spite of this the majority of patients are referred to neurological clinics with the provisional diagnosis of one or the other of these disorders, and the condition is usually referred to in the British literature as 'migrainous neuralgia'.

Cluster headache is considerably less common than migraine. Friedman diagnosed 237 cases of cluster headache and 2667 migrainous patients over a 9 year period. In published series cluster headache varies in incidence from 2–9 per cent of that of migraine.[61]

CLINICAL FEATURES

Sex Incidence

Cluster headache is a notable exception to feminine dominance of the problem of chronic headache. Most series favour males in the ratio of 3–6:1. Of 60 of our patients only 8 were female. The male: female ratio was thus 6·5:1.

Age of Onset

The illness begins in the second and third decades of life in the majority of patients (*Figure 12.1*). In our series of 60 patients,[116] fifteen (25 per cent) started to have attacks between the ages of 16 and 20 years and 35 (68 per cent) between 11 and 30 years. One patient became subject to isolated episodes of retro-orbital pain and lacrimation at the age of 8 years, which recurred twice each year until typical bouts occurred in his second decade. The latest age of onset was 62 years.

Site of Pain

The pain of cluster headache is unilateral, almost always affecting the same side of the head in each bout, although there have been cases reported in which it has changed sides in different bouts. In 32 of our 60 patients, the attacks were exclusively right-sided, in 23 left-sided and in 5 the side affected varied from bout to bout or on different days in the same bout. The pain is felt deeply in and around the eye by about 60 per cent of patients (*Figure 12.2*). It commonly radiates to the supra-orbital region, temple, maxilla and upper gum on the same side of the face. In some patients the ipsilateral nostril aches and burns, and a few complain of aching in the roof of the mouth. In other patients, the lower gum, jaw or chin are also involved. The pain may spread to the ear, the neck or 'the entire half of the head'.

Quality of Pain

The pain of cluster headache is peculiarly distressing. It may be throbbing or pulsating on occasions but the majority describe the pain as constant and severe. Common adjectives used to describe it are

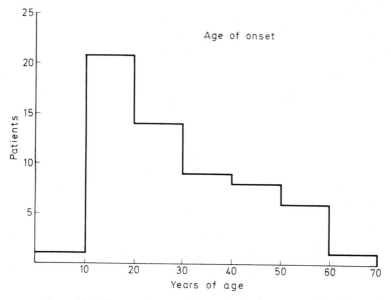

Figure 12.1. The age of onset of cluster headache in 60 patients[116]

burning, boring, piercing, tearing and screwing. One patient stated that it was like a blunt knife being pushed in and turned. Two of our patients said that a dull background pain persisted in the temple or upper jaw between attacks, and 4 patients mentioned a dull ache preceding a bout by some hours or days. Three patients said that they had sometimes experienced sudden jabs of pain in the affected areas at the time of the headache. We have had experience of one patient whose cluster headaches were associated with tic douloureux. A summary of his case history is presented here because of its relevance to a possible neural mechanism for the syndrome.

Case Report

Cluster headache associated with tic douloureux:

A man aged 46 years was well until the age of 42 when he first developed transient shooting, stabbing pains in the inner side of the right lower gum and the adjacent right side of the tongue, which were brought on by movements of the tongue. The pain was severe and initially recurred as single jabs, then as repeated jabs intermittently through the day. After 2 weeks the pain spread to involve the upper gum, and each stab radiated to the midline of the upper and lower jaw. After 3 months each pain seemed to flash up to the right temple and in front of the right temporo-mandibular joint 'as a single hit'.

Site of pain

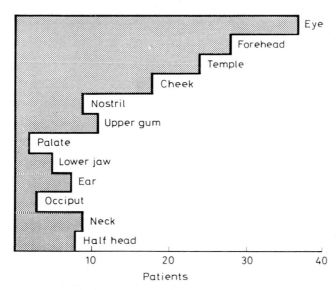

Figure 12.2. The site of pain in 60 patients[116]

Two months later he had his first attack of headache which followed a bad episode of his jabbing pain. On this occasion, pain remained in the right temple for half an hour. The right eye watered, the right nostril ached and discharged a clear fluid. This more prolonged pain lasted for 30 minutes and returned three times daily for some weeks. After 1 month the pain radiated up to the vertex and persisted for 30–90 minutes, recurring 2–3 times daily. After 5 days this variety of pain disappeared but the jabbing pain continued. The jabbing pains were precipitated by swallowing, talking or touching the right lower lip and were stopped by taking carbamazepine 400 mg three times daily.

155

The pain in the temple radiating up to the vertex disappeared for 2 months at a time, would return for 5 days, then again vanish, and recurred in this pattern for 3 years. When the tic-like pain was controlled by carbamazepine, the cluster headache ceased. The tic-like pain, but not the cluster type of pain, recurred after 12 months of treatment with carbamazepine. The second and third divisions of the trigeminal nerve were then sectioned intracranially with complete relief of pain. No abnormality was seen in the Gasserian ganglion or trigeminal nerve at operation.

A similar association has been reported previously by others.[186]

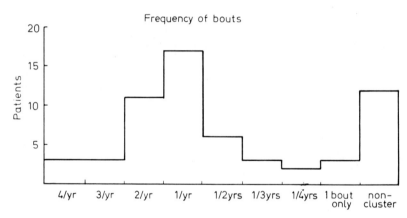

Figure 12.3. The frequency of bouts in 60 patients[116]

Periodicity of Bouts

Cluster headache is so called because of its tendency to recur in bouts or clusters, although about one-fifth of patients with the characteristic pain and accompaniments have a pattern of recurrence which resembles that of migraine without any long periods of freedom. These are designated 'non-cluster' in *Figure 12.3* and are sometimes called chronic cluster headache. Four of our patients were subject to attacks of pain from 1 to 4 times a week without ever having suffered a bout of regular daily episodes. The other 8 of our non-cluster or chronic cluster headache patients had started in this manner but the frequency had increased until they were experiencing from 1 to 5 attacks daily. The remaining patients of our series were subject to bouts with sufficient regularity to enable them to be classified in *Figure 12.3*. Most patients suffered one or two bouts each year.

156

The periodicity of bouts did not depend consistently upon the time of year. Of those who considered that their bouts had a seasonal incidence, 5 stated that they recurred in spring, 6 in summer, 6 in autumn and 7 in winter.

Duration of Bouts

The usual length of each bout is shown in *Figure 12.4*, from 4–8 weeks being the most common. It should be noted that within

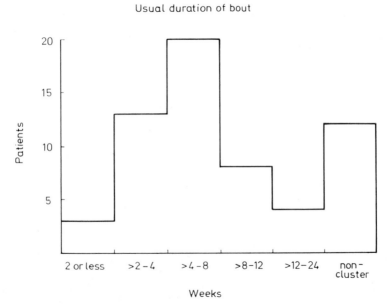

Figure 12.4. The usual duration of each bout in 60 patients[116]

the 'non-cluster' category are included some patients who had been experiencing daily attacks for 12 months without any indication of such a prolonged 'bout' ending.

Daily Frequency of Attacks During a Bout

The usual number of attacks daily is 1–3 as shown in *Figure 12.5*, but the maximum may be 8 or more. The 4 of our patients who had never experienced headaches every day are excluded from *Figure 12.5*.

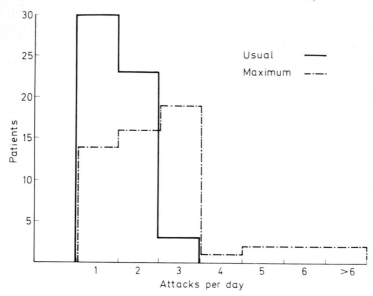

Figure 12.5. The number of attacks experienced per day.[116] *Continuous line, usual frequency; interrupted line, maximum frequency for each patient*

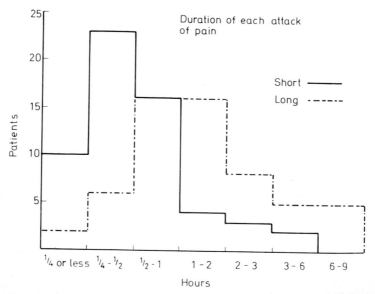

Figure 12.6. The duration of the attacks of pain.[116] *Continuous line, the shortest attacks; interrupted line, the longest attack experienced by each patient*

Of our 60 patients, 52 stated that their attacks were liable to recur at a particular time of the day or night, 32 mentioned 'night time', 9 specifically from 10 p.m. to 2 a.m., and 13 from 2 a.m. to 6 a.m.

Duration of Attacks

Each particular episode usually starts suddenly, lasts for 10 minutes to 2 hours (*Figure 12.6*) and may end abruptly or fade away more slowly.

Associated Features (*Table 12.1*)

Lacrimation from the eye on the affected side is usually the most common symptom and occasionally lacrimation is bilateral. The conjunctiva is often injected on the side of the headache. Drooping of the ipsilateral eyelid and miosis occur in about one-third of patients and may, rarely, persist between attacks (*see Figure 5.1*). Some complain of excessive bilateral sweating during attacks, including patients with ptosis and miosis, indicating that the ocular sympathetic nerve supply is involved discretely. Blurred vision may be noticed in the ipsilateral eye, which cannot be attributed to excessive lacrimation since some do not have this symptom.

The nostril is often blocked or running on one or both sides. A running nostril cannot be explained by lacrimation in all cases since it is not always associated with a weeping eye.

Gastrointestinal disturbances are less common than in migraine but about one-half the patients feel nauseated and may vomit. Two of our patients were certain that nausea preceded the onset of facial pain on each occasion.

Vascular phenomena are particularly interesting. The superficial temporal artery on the affected side may become prominent, more than usually pulsatile, and tender to touch; superficial veins may dilate. Four of our patients stated that their pain was relieved by compressing the temporal artery, although one emphasized that pain still persisted deep to the eye. Facial flushing is more common than pallor and was the origin of the old term 'red migraine'.

Hyperalgesia of the face and scalp is common and can be extreme in some cases so that the patient cannot bear to touch the affected areas. Two of our patients had noticed an itching sensation behind the eye, one immediately preceding pain in the eye and the other for some weeks before a bout began.

Focal neurological symptoms or signs, of the type which are common in migraine, are unusual in cluster headache. One of our patients mentioned occasional 'spots before the eyes' and another

TABLE 12.1
ASSOCIATED FEATURES IN 60 PATIENTS[116]

Ocular	
lacrimation { unilateral	49
{ bilateral	3
conjunctival injection	27
partial Horner's syndrome	19
photophobia	12
blurred vision	5
Nasal	
blocked nostril { unilateral	28
{ bilateral	4
running nostril { unilateral	9
{ bilateral	1
epistaxis	1
Gastrointestinal	
anorexia	2
nausea	26
vomiting { occasionally	9
{ regularly	8
diarrhoea	2
Vascular	
flushing of face	12
pallor of face	2
prominent, tender temporal artery	10
prominent veins in forehead	2
puffiness around eyes	6
lumps in mouth	2
cold hands and feet	1
polyuria	4
Neurological	
hyperalgesia of scalp and face	10
itching behind eye (preceding headache)	2
flashing lights in front of eyes	1
spots in front of eyes	1
vertigo and mild ataxia	4
mental confusion	1
unilateral carpal spasm	1

described 'little flashing lights in front of the eyes' during the head-ache. Four described a feeling of dizziness, giddiness, or a 'rising feeling in the head' associated with impaired balance at the time of the attack. One patient had experienced a tonic seizure of the left arm on three occasions associated with a pain in the right eye and temple. The left hand assumed the position of carpal spasm for a period of minutes. Sutherland and Eadie reported a patient who was subject to scintillating scotomata before cluster headache, two patients with paraesthesiae on the side of the body opposite to the head pain, and one patient with twitching of the contralateral foot.

Precipitating Factors

The only trigger factor which is consistently mentioned by patients is the taking of alcoholic drinks and this is only operative during a susceptible period, that is to say, during a bout. Other vasodilator substances have been used experimentally to precipitate an attack. One of our patients who used carbon tetrachloride as a solvent in his daily work commented that inhalation of the fumes would induce an attack as readily as alcohol. Other factors mentioned by patients are stress, attacks of hay fever, heat, changes in weather, glare, missing a meal or sleeping late in the mornings.

Relieving Factors

Some patients can find some ease from their pain by pressing on the superficial temporal arteries, by the application of heat, or by pacing up and down with their hand clasped over one eye.

PAST HISTORY

There is nothing very remarkable in the past health of patients with cluster headache and no convincing association with migraine or allergic disorders.

Migraine

Four of our 60 patients had been subject to frequent vomiting attacks in childhood and there was a history of migraine in 4 patients, one of whom continued to have occasional migraine headaches between bouts of cluster headache.

Allergy

Of 60 patients, 9 had suffered from allergic disorders, 2 from hives, 2 from asthma, 4 from hay fever and 1 from both asthma and hay fever. Two patients were of particular interest in that bouts of cluster headache regularly followed 2–4 weeks after episodes of hay fever. One of these patients stated that his hay fever was becoming milder each year but that his bouts of cluster headache were becoming longer and more severe. Allergy tests were performed in 4 patients, 1 of whom had a history of hives, but no positive skin test was obtained.

Trauma

Eight of our 60 patients had experienced a head injury, and in 4 the site of injury could conceivably be relevant to the ensuing cluster headache. One patient had required extensive plastic surgery

161

for facial and scalp lacerations following a car accident and left-sided cluster headache started 21 months after injury. The second had gravel embedded in the right temple from a road accident at the age of 17 years and cluster headaches involving the right temple and right side of the face began 7 years later. The third patient developed right frontotemporal cluster headache 30 years after a shotgun injury to the forehead, in which fragmented pellets were still embedded. The fourth patient experienced a blow on the forehead at the age of 22 years, following which he was subject to a dull right-sided head-ache for 3 years. Eight years after the injury, right-sided cluster headaches developed, involving the right forehead and right side of the face.

Other Illnesses of Possible Relevance

Disorders worthy of note in our series were meningitis 7 years before the onset of cluster headache, right-sided stapedectomy 6 months before the onset of right-sided cluster headache, excessive lacrimation of the right eye without obvious ocular cause for 3 years before bouts of pain in the right eye started, and loss of pinprick and temperature sensation over the right side of the neck and right arm in a man of 52, 6 years before right-sided cluster headache began. One female patient suffered from chronic lymphatic leukaemia, and one male patient had required treatment for a depressive state.

FAMILY HISTORY

Of our 60 patients, 13 had a family history of migraine affecting a parent or sibling. None had any member of the family afflicted by cluster headache. The incidence of migraine in parents and siblings (22 per cent in our series) is not significantly greater than that of patients with tension headache (18 per cent) and much less than that of typical migrainous patients (45 per cent).[113] Ekbom[61] found a family history of migraine in 16 per cent of patients with cluster headache compared with 65 per cent of migrainous patients. It is rare to find other examples of cluster headache in the family history. Examples have been cited by Bickerstaff,[21] Nieman and Hurwitz,[138] Balla and Walton,[15] Sutherland and Eadie,[186] and Ekbom.[61]

PATHOPHYSIOLOGY

IS THIS SYNDROME A VARIANT OF MIGRAINE?

The common denominator of both migraine and cluster headache is dilatation of the extracranial arteries, although this is strictly unilateral

162

in cluster headache and tends to become bilateral in migraine. The internal carotid artery is also involved in most patients with cluster headache as judged by the frequency of retro-orbital pain and of paralysis of the ocular sympathetic supply, which most authorities agree is caused by compression of the sympathetic plexus in the carotid canal by distension of the wall of the internal carotid artery.[109,138] The localization of the lesion in the sympathetic pathway is aided by the sparing of facial sweating, which is mediated by the sympathetic plexus surrounding extracranial vessels.

Kunkle *et al.*[110] injected normal saline intrathecally under pressure without benefit in 2 patients, but these patients had responded to ergotamine tartrate, suggesting that arterial vasodilatation was mainly extracranial in their cases. The dual source of pain in cluster headache, intracranial and extracranial, is illustrated by one of our patients who found that he could relieve the pain in his temple by compressing his dilated superficial temporal artery, but that some pain persisted, felt deeply behind the eye. Ekbom and Greitz[62a] recently reported vascular changes demonstrated by angiography during an episode of cluster headache. At the height of the attack, the internal carotid artery showed localized narrowing after emerging from the carotid canal; this was attributed to oedema or spasm and persisted after pain had ceased. In contrast, the ophthalmic artery was dilated during the attack.

The importance of vascular dilatation in cluster headache is emphasized by the ease with which headaches may be triggered during a bout by vasodilators such as alcohol, histamine[94a] and nitroglycerin,[61] and their prevention by the prophylactic use of ergotamine tartrate[189] or regular medication with methysergide.[47]

One important difference between the vascular changes of migraine and cluster headache is that the majority of patients become pale in migraine because of constriction of cutaneous capillaries, whereas this is uncommon in cluster headache (2 out of 60 in our series). On the contrary, 12 of our patients (20 per cent) noticed flushing of face. Horton[94a] noted that skin temperatures were 1–3 degC higher on the side of the headache. Recent thermographic studies[115] demonstrated an increase of skin temperature over the painful area in only 3 of the 5 patients studied (Plate 1). Two of these patients showed a 'cold spot' over the eye on the affected side in the early phase of headache (Plate 1) which is very similar to the cold area observed on the forehead of patients with stenosis or occlusion of the internal carotid artery because of inadequate filling of the terminal branches of the ophthalmic artery which supply the skin of the forehead. Broch *et al.*[31] have reported that blood flow in the internal carotid artery was unaltered in 3 patients during cluster headache, so that the mechanism of the cool forehead cannot be explained by constriction of the lumen of the carotid artery. It is possible that flow in the ophthalmic artery reverses during the early stages of cluster headache or that its cutaneous branches are constricted. At a later stage of the headache, the temperature of the forehead and affected areas increases in most patients. The frequency of conjunctival injection and nasal blockage in cluster headache supports the view that facial and scalp capillaries dilate. This may be associated with oedema, causing swelling of the periorbital region or buccal mucosa.

TABLE 12.2

DIFFERENCES BETWEEN MIGRAINE AND 'CLUSTER HEADACHE'[116]

	Migraine	Cluster headache
Sex incidence (%)	female 75	male 85
Onset in childhood (%)	25	< 1
Unilateral pain (%)	65	100
Recurrence in bouts (%)	0	80
Frequency of attacks	< 1–12/month	1–8/day
Usual duration of pain	4–24 h	0·25–2 h
Associated features:		
nausea, vomiting (%)	85	45
blurring of vision (%)	common	8
lacrimation (%)	uncommon	85
blocked nostril (%)	uncommon	50
ptosis, miosis (%)	uncommon	25
hyperalgesia of face, scalp (%)	65	15
teichopsia, photopsia (%)	40	< 1
polyuria (%)	30	7
Past health:		
vomiting in childhood (%)	25	7
Family history:		
migraine (%)	50	20
Biochemical changes:		
fall in plasma serotonin (%)	80	0
rise in plasma histamine (%)	0	90
rise in CSF acetylcholine (%)	0	30

Visual disturbance, such as zig-zags of light (fortification spectra, teichopsia) or unformed flashes of light (photopsia) are very common in migraine, affecting 30–40 per cent of patients before or during the headache,[113,166] but are very rare in cluster headache.

Considering the vascular phenomena of migraine and cluster headache, the following tentative comparison may be drawn. In migraine, vessels supplying the cerebral cortex often constrict, some large intracranial arteries may dilate,[108] extracranial arteries dilate and scalp and facial capillaries usually constrict. In cluster headache, the ophthalmic artery, extracranial arteries and scalp and facial capillaries all usually dilate, while the lumen of the internal carotid artery is narrowed.

There are many other factors which distinguish cluster headache from migraine, such as the predominantly male incidence, the pattern of recurrence and the brief duration of pain. These are listed in Table 12.2 which has been prepared from various publications.[11,61,113,116,166] The only factor in common between migraine and the syndrome under discussion is the dilatation of the extracranial arteries which has been observed at the height of the attack, and the relief of pain by drugs which constrict these vessels or prevent their dilatation. In every other respect, clinical and biochemical, the disorders differ, as outlined in Table 12.2. Apart from an occasional unexplained association with tic douloureux, there is no evidence that the condition has a neuralgic basis. It is therefore suggested that the misleading designation 'migrainous neuralgia' be replaced by the descriptive term 'cluster headache', until such time as the aetiology is fully understood. Exception can be taken to the use of 'cluster headache' on the grounds that about one-fifth of patients do not experience the typical periodicity of attacks implied by the name but the term is already accepted in medical literature and is more succinct and expressive than any alternative.

Is This Syndrome of Humoral Origin?

Cluster headache is thus characterized by periodic vascular instability which is only rarely familial. If there is a primary disorder of humoral control of blood vessels, which chemical agents are involved? The syndrome is consistent with an excessive discharge of cholinergic nerve endings and it is of interest that Kunkle[107] demonstrated an acetylcholine effect from cerebrospinal fluid specimens taken at the time of headache in 4 out of 14 patients with cluster headache which was not present in 7 patients with typical migraine. Plasma serotonin has been shown to fall during migraine headache,[7,45] but does not alter significantly at the time of cluster headache.[11]

Since the reports by Horton and his colleagues, histamine has been considered as a possible mediator of cluster headache, although antihistaminic agents are not of value in treatment and the place of histamine desensitization is still controversial. Recently, Anthony and Lance[11] reported that the mean blood level of histamine increased during cluster headache from 0·045 to 0·053 $\mu g/ml$ ($P < 0·001$), but did not alter significantly in migraine headache. This finding

165

differentiates cluster headache from migraine on biochemical as well as clinical grounds and renews interest in the possibility that histamine release plays some part in the symptomatology of cluster headache. It is tempting to think of the thickening of the wall of the internal carotid artery, which has been shown radiographically, as carotid 'hives' which causes intense pain by distension of the wall and compresses the pericarotid sympathetic plexus.

Is this Syndrome of Neural Origin?

A neurogenic mechanism has been considered because of the sudden onset of pain, its brief duration and the association with lacrimation and blockage of the nostril.

Stimulation of the parasympathetic fibres travelling via the greater superficial petrosal nerve to the sphenopalatine ganglion evokes lacrimation and rhinorrhoea,[156] but transection of the greater superficial petrosal nerve has not prevented patients from having further attacks. White and Sweet[209] stimulated the greater superficial petrosal nerve during craniotomy under local anaesthesia in 14 patients. Nine patients experienced pain localized to the ear, eye or adjacent parts of the head or face. After section of the nerve, pain could be elicited by stimulation of the central end only, indicating that the effect was mediated through afferent fibres and not indirectly by peripheral vasodilatation. The nerve was divided in 6 patients with cluster headache, but all experienced recurrence of pain at varying intervals postoperatively.

The stellate ganglion was blocked in 2 of our patients during a bout, producing a Horner's syndrome, but not provoking an attack. This suggests that a deficiency of sympathetic activity is not the primary factor. There have been no reports of any surgical operation preventing further bouts of cluster headache, although section of trigeminal nerve will relieve the painful component of the attack arising from areas which it supplies.

In many instances pain involves the occipital area, neck or ear, areas supplied by the second and third cervical spinal segments. It is known that afferent fibres from the upper three cervical nerve roots make synaptic contact with neurones of the spinal nucleus of the trigeminal nerve in the upper cervical cord.[103] It is therefore theoretically possible for a disturbance in this area to cause pain of both trigeminal and upper cervical distribution. A syndrome resembling cluster headache has been reported following whiplash injury to the neck in 8 patients.[96] Of our 60 patients 8 had experienced head injuries and the site of facial injury bore some relationship to the site of cluster headache in 4 patients. It is possible that injury to central or peripheral nervous pathways could cause vessels in the area of defective neurogenic control to become more susceptible to the action of humoral agents such as histamine. In view of male proneness to injury, this could explain why cluster headache is predominantly a male disease whereas migraine and tension headache are more common in women.

TREATMENT

The pain of cluster headache is so intense that patients understandably become apprehensive about the arrival of the next attack and may become depressed if their pain is not controlled. The effectiveness of treatment is difficult to assess because of possible variations in the length of each bout. Histamine desensitization was advocated before the natural history of the disorder was fully understood, so that a spontaneous remission was interpreted as a success for the treatment. The author has encountered patients who claimed that previous bouts had been stopped by histamine desensitization but who failed to gain relief when the same regimen was undertaken at the beginning of the next bout. With the recent demonstration of histamine release at the time of cluster headache, the value of antihistaminic agents must be reassessed. Failure of these agents in the past may have been related to their inability to counteract the action of tissue-bound histamine. There have been recent reports of pizotifen (BC105, Sandomigran), a potent antihistamine and antiserotonin agent, preventing further attacks of pain when taken in the dose of two 0·5 mg tablets three times daily during a bout.

In the absence of further knowledge of the mechanism of cluster headache, the most useful treatment is to attack one of the manifestations which gives rise to pain, dilatation of the extracranial arteries. The agents used are the same as for migraine but must be given regularly once, twice or three times each day, depending upon the times of the day when an attack of pain would be expected. In milder cases, oral preparations containing ergotamine tartrate such as Gynergen or Cafergot may be given as two tablets night and morning, or a Cafergot suppository may be inserted on retiring to bed if the attacks are solely nocturnal. If this fails, ergotamine tartrate 0·5 mg can be given by intramuscular injection at night, or twice daily, or methysergide can be administered orally in a dose of 2 mg three times daily. In some patients with severe cluster headache I have increased the dose of methysergide gradually to 12–15 mg daily before relief has been obtained. Provided the patient does not experience any side-effects (discussed in Chapter 11) as the dose is being increased, a high dosage of methysergide may be continued for the duration of the bout without cause for concern. As the anticipated end of the bout approaches, treatment should be ceased for a day to assess whether it is necessary to continue or not. If a characteristic attack ensues, then treatment is continued for another week before another test day of abstinence from medication. I have found methysergide and injected ergotamine tartrate each to be effective in about 70 per cent of patients.

The patients who continue to have attacks of severe pain in spite of these treatments present a very difficult problem. Carbamazepine (Tegretol) is occasionally useful. A trial of progesterone and corticosteroids has been suggested but my limited experience with this has not been encouraging. Section of the appropriate divisions of the trigeminal nerve may have to be considered if the patient is subject to frequent and intense bouts which are not relieved by other means.

13—The Investigation and Management of Headache Problems

When you're lying awake with a dismal headache,
and repose is taboo'd by anxiety,
I conceive you may use any language you choose
To indulge in, without impropriety.

Iolanthe, *W. S. Gilbert*

A headache, at best, is an unpleasant thing. It is more unpleasant because it attacks the seat of reason, and there are few patients with headache who are not troubled by thoughts of cerebral tumour or intracranial disaster. For the doctor to be able to reassure his patient, he must have a clear idea of the diagnosis, based on clinical judgment and supported when necessary by special investigations.

The initial problem in management is the decision as to whether any special investigation is warranted. In the majority of patients, a careful history will establish the pattern so clearly that any special tests are superfluous. When there is diagnostic difficulty or when the history suggests a serious disorder, investigation becomes obligatory, and judgment is required to determine the sequence of tests which is safest for the patient and most likely to produce a definitive answer.

The clinical approach will depend upon the duration of headache and its mode of presentation.

The Acute Severe Headache

When a headache suddenly develops in a patient for the first time, the presence or absence of fever and neck rigidity is of great importance. Patients with acute headache, photophobia, elevation of body temperature and neck stiffness obviously have an intracranial disturbance, and the question of lumbar puncture arises. If there are other signs of one of the infectious fevers then lumbar puncture can be deferred. The CSF commonly shows a lymphocytic pleocytosis

169

if headache is present at the height of a viral invasion but this knowledge does not assist in management. When a confident diagnosis of a specific infection cannot be made after examination of the patient, lumbar puncture may be necessary to distinguish between meningitis, encephalitis and subarachnoid haemorrhage. The normal CSF should not contain more than 5 lymphocytes/mm^3 and should never contain polymorphonuclear cells. A high polymorph count is almost always caused by bacterial meningitis and a purely lymphocytic reaction indicates a viral meningoencephalitis, but mixed cellular reactions may be found in both viral and bacterial infections, particularly in tuberculous meningitis. The glucose content of CSF assumes particular significance in these doubtful cases. The CSF level of glucose depends upon the blood level but, providing that the patient is not hypoglycaemic and that the fluid has not been allowed to stand for some hours before examination, a CSF glucose of 30 mg/100 ml or less suggests a bacterial or cryptococcal meningitis, or the rare meningitis carcinomatosa.

Apart from the diagnosis of infectious disease, lumbar puncture may be required to confirm the diagnosis of subarachnoid haemorrhage. If the diagnosis of subarachnoid haemorrhage is self-evident and the patient is conscious, it is often better to proceed immediately to cerebral angiography in a centre which is suitably equipped, since lumbar puncture gives no additional information and may precipitate further bleeding.

After head injury, there may be difficulty in distinguishing post-concussional vascular headache from that of an expanding intracranial haematoma. A unilateral headache and insidious drowsiness are always signals to be on the alert. Dilatation of one pupil or a minimal hemiparesis are late signs which should prompt immediate carotid angiography and neurosurgical intervention. Neck stiffness arising in this context is a particular source of concern as it suggests mid-brain compression from 'coning' of one temporal lobe through the tentorial opening. When radiography of the skull demonstrates a fracture of the lateral aspect, the possibility of an extradural haematoma from a torn middle meningeal artery should be borne in mind, and justifies close observation of the patient. An electroencephalogram (EEG) or brain scan is also helpful in following the course of patients with a post-traumatic headache of doubtful origin.

Acute headaches without neck stiffness may also be of intracranial origin. Blood pressure may suddenly increase in acute nephritis, toxaemia of pregnancy, malignant hypertension, and the crises caused by phaeochromocytoma or by a patient on mono-amine oxidase inhibitors taking sympathomimetic drugs or tyramine-containing foods. The latter syndrome will probably become more common with the increasing use of MAO inhibitors for depression. The finding of hypertension on examination does not of course mean that the patient does not have an intracranial lesion as the source of headache. The blood pressure is usually secondarily elevated in patients with subarachnoid and intracerebral haemorrhage.

Acute headaches of extracranial origin (sinusitis, retrobulbar neuritis, acute angle-closure glaucoma and abscesses around the roots of the upper teeth) can usually be diagnosed clinically.

Acute Recurrent Episodes of Headaches

Some of the entities mentioned above (sinusitis, pressor reaction of phaeochromocytoma) may recur periodically. Repeated episodes of meningitis suggest either defective immunological mechanisms or, more commonly, that the nasopharynx communicates with the subarachnoid space through a fracture in the floor of the anterior fossa. This leads to CSF rhinorrhoea, with clear fluid dripping from the nostril when the head is bent forwards. CSF, unlike nasal secretions, contains glucose so that a Clinistix dipped into the nostril can rapidly confirm that the fluid is of intracranial origin. The fistula can be repaired surgically with a fascial graft.

Repetition of subarachnoid haemorrhage from intracranial aneurysm carries a mortality in the vicinity of 50 per cent, like that of the original episode. Cerebral, cerebellar or spinal angiomas on the other hand may bleed 'little and often' throughout life, with little or no residual deficit. Angiomas can be dealt with surgically if their arterial supply is accessible, but in other cases any surgical procedure could cause more havoc than the natural history of the disease, so that the patient is advised to ride out each storm as it comes.

Attacks of cerebrovascular insufficiency are clearly demarcated by symptoms and signs of the territory which is rendered ischaemic. The classical story of internal carotid insufficiency, usually seen only in part, is that of blurring of vision in one eye (resulting from retinal ischaemia) accompanied by fleeting paraesthesiae or paresis of the opposite side. If the dominant hemisphere (the left in right-handed subjects; either or both in left-handed patients) is involved, dysphasia is an additional symptom. Transient ischaemic attacks may be accompanied by headache on the side supplied by the defective carotid artery. Insufficiency of the vertebrobasilar artery is characterized by momentary vertigo, dysarthria and ataxia, or by a mélange of brainstem symptoms and signs, including diplopia, tinnitus, deafness, paraesthesiae over the face and body and hemiparesis or quadriparesis. Because the posterior cerebral arteries, which supply the occipital cortex, arise from the basilar artery, the patient may experience a temporary homonymous hemianopia, visual hallucinations like those of migraine, or a complete bilateral suppression of vision. Since the medial part of the temporal lobe, which is the entry portal of the brain for memory, is also within the distribution of the posterior cerebral artery, amnesia may also be a feature of vertebro-basilar attacks. The occipital headache, which may be present for the duration of the attack, is insignificant compared with the dramatic nature of the focal neurological symptoms.

The investigation of cerebral vascular insufficiency is beyond the scope of this book, but it is worth emphasizing that the history and examination may indicate the underlying cause of the attacks. Paroxysmal cardiac dysrhythmias may produce the attacks through hypotension, sudden neck movements may obliterate the lumen of the vertebral artery in the neck of spondylitic patients, and arm movements may induce a shunting of blood from the vertebral artery into the subclavian artery if its intraluminal pressure is lowered because of stenosis in the first part of the vessel. Inequality of the radial pulses and a bruit over the clavicles or in the neck may indicate the site of stenoses in major vessels.

Intermittent hydrocephalus is a rare cause of recurrent headache, but should be considered if the history is relatively short, if the headaches are severe, if they are precipitated by a quick forward movement of the head, or are associated with obscuration of vision, impairment of consciousness, myoclonic jerks or weakness of the legs. The final diagnosis will depend upon carotid angiography and air studies.

The pattern of pain or headache in tic douloureux, cluster headache and migraine has been considered at some length earlier in this book and is usually sufficiently distinctive for a diagnosis to be made (*Figure 13.1*). Where doubt exists, other conditions may be excluded by investigations, but a positive diagnosis depends upon the clinical story. The diagnosis of migraine is supported by the finding of a low plasma level of serotonin at the time of a headache. This cannot be used as a routine test for migraine because most laboratories do not estimate serotonin often enough for accurate results to be obtained, and because plasma serotonin varies so much between individuals that a baseline level has to be established for that particular patient before the level in the headache samples can be interpreted.

Migraine may be accompanied by any of the symptoms which were mentioned in the description of cerebral vascular insufficiency. Indeed, these features of migraine may be regarded as a prolonged ischaemia of internal carotid or vertebrobasilar territory as the result of arterial vasoconstriction. The duration of focal neurological symptoms in migraine commonly varies from 10 to 30 minutes, but there are instances in which they may be prolonged for hours or days, or keep recurring intermittently for weeks, as 'status migrainosus vasospasticus'. One patient aged 26 years has experienced several episodes of recurring bilateral scintillating scotomas and left homonymous hemianopia lasting up to 2 weeks, associated with numbness, weakness and continuous epileptic jerking of the left side of the body on one occasion, and dysarthria, dyscoordination of the right hand, ataxia and stupor on another. Residual deficits have taken some months to resolve. The associated headache has been unilateral, commonly left-sided. It is only after years of observation and repeated investigations that this syndrome can confidently be regarded as a variant of migraine.

The fact that different areas of brain or brainstem have been involved on different occasions, that the headache has varied from right to left, and that the headache has at times been on the side inappropriate for the initiation of the focal symptoms, all favour the diagnosis of migraine, and may be helpful in assessing symptoms which could be caused either by migrainous vasospasm or by a fixed intracranial lesion.

Headache of Subacute Onset

This group is of interest to the doctor and of potential danger to the patient. Someone who has never experienced more than 'ordinary headaches' which most of us get at times, starts to complain of a different sort of headache which may affect one or both sides and becomes progressively more severe. If the patient has been complaining of earache, or of nasal obstruction with pain over the forehead or maxillae before the onset of headache, thoughts turn to the intracranial complications of otitis media and sinusitis.

If the patient has signs of raised intracranial pressure, the EEG is very useful in deciding whether a focal lesion such as a cerebral abscess is present (*see Figure 7.4*). When the EEG is nonspecific, a carotid angiogram will determine whether the lateral ventricles are large or small (*see Figure 6.6*). If the lateral ventricles are not enlarged and there is no displacement of vessels, it is safe to introduce air through a lumbar puncture needle to delineate the ventricular system by pneumoencephalography. If the ventricles are large there is probably an obstructive hydrocephalus and it is safer for a neurosurgeon to drain the lateral ventricles and later find the site of obstruction by injecting air or a radio-opaque substance into the ventricular system (*see Figure 6.7*).

The rare case of Addison's disease or hypocalcaemia presenting with increased intracranial pressure must be remembered and excluded.

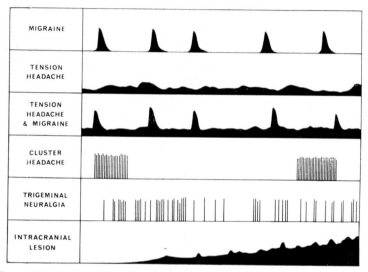

Figure 13.1. Temporal patterns of headache discussed in Chapter 4. This scheme does not bring out the difference in duration between the pain of trigeminal neuralgia (repeated jabs lasting a fraction of a second) and that of cluster headache (each lasting 20 to 120 minutes)

Electroencephalography and brain scanning are also of great assistance when tumour or subdural haematoma is suspected. The EEG is abnormal in the majority of patients with these conditions and can indicate the probable side and position of the lesion in most cases so that carotid arteriography can be done on the appropriate side. The brain scan may outline precisely the site of tumour or haematoma.

In patients over the age of 55 years the blood picture and erythrocyte sedimentation rate should always be examined to pick up the odd patient with temporal arteritis.

Chronic Headache

In the patient who has suffered from headaches for a year or more, the prospect of a tumour or other serious intracranial disorder being the cause is more remote, but one cannot be completely sure unless the duration of the patient's headaches is more than 5 years. If the patient's headaches have been consistent in character for 5 years or more one may feel fairly confident that they are not caused by intracranial tumour, although the occasional patient may be found to have a tumour which is quite unrelated to the headache with which they presented. The author recalls a patient with a pituitary tumour who complained of a typical tension headache, which responded well to treatment in spite of its duration of 20 years. The author missed the significance of her appearance and did not investigate further. Some time later she presented with bilateral carpal tunnel syndrome, induced by acromegaly, when the diagnosis of pituitary tumour was finally made. The author remains convinced that her headache was not caused by her tumour.

Of the 1,152 patients who attended a clinic for chronic headache, only 1 was found to have a cerebral tumour. The diagnosis was made by finding intracranial calcification on radiography of the skull, which was done to reassure the patient, whose symptoms were those of tension headache.

As a general rule, any headache which has been present for more than 5 years is a muscle-contraction headache or migraine.

THE INVESTIGATION OF HEADACHE

Only a small percentage of patients with headache requires any investigation other than a careful history and examination.

Blood Count and Erythrocyte Sedimentation Rate (ESR)

These are routine tests for patients admitted to hospital and should be done in general practice when there have been symptoms of systemic disorder, or signs of infection or meningeal reaction associated with headache, or in a patient above the age of 55 years in whom the possibility of temporal arteritis must be ruled out. Polycythaemia may be the result of arteriovenous shunting as in cerebral angioma, haemangioblastoma of the cerebellum and Paget's disease. Leukaemia may present with intracranial deposits. Anaemia may indicate neoplasia or other systemic disease, and may accentuate any tendency to headache. A high ESR often directs attention to some locus of infection, hidden malignancy or an unusual condition such as myelomatosis, one of the collagen diseases or sub-acute bacterial endocarditis, which may all produce intracranial manifestations.

Lumbar Puncture

Some recent medical graduates assume that a lumbar puncture must be done in any patient complaining of neurological symptoms, and await each new admission with needle poised. If there were such a concept as a 'routine neurological work-up', which fortunately there is not, lumbar puncture would not usually form part of it. There are specific indications for lumbar puncture, and suspected intracranial tumour is not one of them. If there is genuine suspicion of cerebral tumour, EEG, brain scan and contrast radiographic studies will be necessary to attempt to localize or exclude it. A sample of CSF can then be taken at the beginning of pneumo-encephalography, although really it helps little to know whether fluid constituents, such as protein, vary slightly from normal. Lumbar puncture is used in the investigation of headache to confirm the presence of subarachnoid haemorrhage, to investigate infectious processes of the nervous system, including syphilis, or to measure intracranial pressure in benign intracranial hypertension.

There is a modern tendency to decry the hazards of lumbar puncture in the presence of papilloedema, but it is potentially dangerous unless preliminary carotid angiography has shown that there is no displacement of intracranial vessels or internal hydro-cephalus. Should lumbar puncture have to be done without this safeguard in a patient with raised intracranial pressure, in, for example, a patient with bilateral papilloedema who is suspected of having bacterial meningitis, it is a worthwhile precaution to have a 20 ml syringe filled with normal saline solution which can be injected intrathecally should any untoward symptoms follow the with-drawal of CSF.

A small point concerning the technique of lumbar puncture which the author has found useful, is to infiltrate the skin with local anaesthetic 1–2 cm laterally to the midline at the selected interverte-bral disc space and to angulate the lumbar puncture needle towards the midline as it is inserted from this point. The suggested track passes through soft tissues until the needle touches the spine. A gentle tapping movement of the needle will indicate to the examiner whether the needle is in contact with bone or with the elastic inter-laminar ligament. If the latter, the needle can be inserted through the ligament with confidence that CSF will emerge when the stilette is removed. The advantages of this lateral approach is that it is usually painless and permits tactile sensibility of the position of the needle point. These advantages are lost with the firm pressure required to penetrate the interspinous ligament in the midline approach, making it difficult to know when the lumbar sac is entered.

Electroencephalography

The EEG can give only a limited range of answers to any clinical question, but is a most useful investigation because it is painless, harmless and relatively inexpensive. It may give a complete answer in some conditions such as intracranial abscess, which gives rise to an angry focus of slow waves (*see Figure 7.4*). It may also give an accurate localization in cerebral tumour, but regrettably the most striking EEG foci are produced by the most rapidly growing and malignant tumours, and a benign tumour of long-standing, such as a meningioma, may not alter the tracing at all. Lateralizing abnormalities may indicate a lesion such as subdural haematoma which interferes with the recording of the normal electrical activity of the brain and induces slow rhythms from the surrounding area of the brain which is compressed. The changes produced by diffuse disorders, such as meningitis, encephalitis, or metabolic disturbances are of little diagnostic value. It is generally agreed that the proportion of abnormal tracings found in migraine is higher than in the general population, but the changes are non-specific and are of no help in diagnosis. The EEG is most useful in the patient whose headaches do not fit any particular pattern, as a partial reassurance against the presence of a space-occupying lesion; or in the patient who is suspected of harbouring such a lesion but has no lateralizing symptoms or signs, as a preliminary to special radiographic investigations. The EEG may give a clear indication of the side of the lesion, and thus guide the clinician as to the side to be examined by carotid angiography. It may also be of indirect benefit in patients with tension headache by disclosing muscle artefact which persists over the site of muscle contraction (*Figure 13.2*).

Plain Radiography

The patient whose headache is sufficiently troublesome to warrant radiography of the skull should always have a film of the chest taken at the same time. There are many ways in which diseases of the heart and lungs may affect the brain. Pulmonary tuberculosis

177

may be associated with tuberculous meningitis, bronchiectasis with cerebral abscess and carcinoma of the lung with cerebral metastases.

Radiography of the skull is an essential stage in the diagnosis of headaches which do not fit into a recognizable benign pattern.

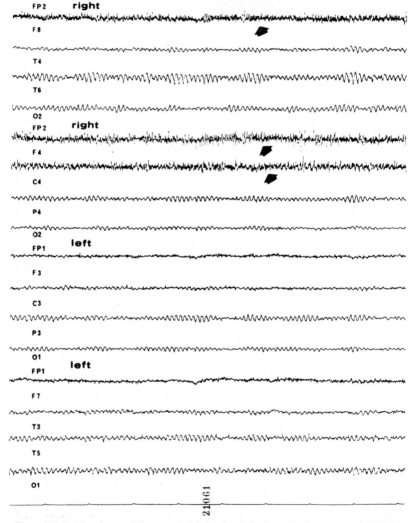

Figure 13.2. Muscle artefact recorded from the right frontal electrodes in a patient with persistent headache over the right frontotemporal region

178

The pituitary fossa is first inspected in the lateral films and then the vault is surveyed systematically, looking for fractures, areas of radiolucency or sclerosis. The angle which the horizontal plane of the axis makes with the hard palate is examined to ensure that there is no platybasia (basilar impression), which has been illustrated in *Figure 6.9*.

Calcification is noted in the normal sites: pineal gland and habenular trigone, choroid plexuses and petro-clinoid ligaments. Abnormal calcification is sought, particularly above the pituitary fossa, the common site for craniopharyngioma. The sinuses and mastoid air cells are inspected. The shadow of the pharyngeal tissue is examined if the question of nasopharyngeal carcinoma has arisen.

In the antero-posterior projections, the position of the pineal gland, if calcified, is checked and any displacement from the midline noted. Any abnormal calcification is localized. The sphenoid wings and the posterior clinoid processes are examined. The sinuses are again examined. In the Towne's view, the internal auditory meatus can be seen clearly on each side. If the patient has a nerve deafness then Stenver's views or tomography of the internal auditory meatus are essential. The basal view of the skull should be searched for fractures, erosions, enlargement of the jugular foramen, foramen ovale or foramen spinosum. The latter may enlarge on the same side as a vascular meningioma because it is traversed by the middle meningeal artery.

Opinions differ about the significance of certain findings. Hyperostosis frontalis interna is regarded by some European authors as an inflammatory condition producing headache. It is a common variation of normal from middle age onwards, particularly in female patients, and the author is unaware of any controlled observations linking it with headache. 'Thumbing', a beaten-copper appearance of the cranial vault, may be a normal variation, although it alerts the observer to the possibility of long-standing raised intracranial pressure (*see Figure 6.9*). The sutures should be observed carefully in the young child as they separate when intracranial pressure is increased.

In most patients with headache, the appearance of the skull radiograph will be normal but a surprise turns up often enough to make the procedure worthwhile (*Figure 13.3*). The most useful facet of skull radiography is often the position of the pineal gland. It must be remembered, however, that midline structures are not always displaced by cerebral tumour, and that a pineal gland remains central with bilateral symmetrical subdural haematomas.

TABLE 13.1
TABLE FOR DIFFERENTIAL DIAGNOSIS OF HEADACHE

	Site	Photo-phobia	Neck Stiffness	Worse on Jolting	Drowsi-ness	Other Focal Symptoms and Signs	EEG	Skull Radiograph	CSF	Arteriogram and PEG
ACUTE SINGLE EPISODES (minutes or hours)										
Subarachnoid haem.	1	+	+	+	+	cer. or b.s.	occ. focal	−	blood-stained	aneurysm angioma
Encephalitis	1	+	+	+	+	cer. or b.s.	nonspec.	−	mainly lympho-cytic	−
Meningitis	1	+	+	+	+	−	nonspec.	−	mainly p.m.n.	−
Post-concussion	1	+	−	+	transient					
Post-traumatic Compression	½ or 1	+ or −	if coning	+	+	c.n.3 ½ paresis	nonspec. usually lateralizing	often skull fracture + pineal shift	L.P. dangerous	extra- or subdural haematoma
Pressor reaction	1	−	−	+	−	−	nonspec.	−	−	−
Systemic Infections	½ or 1	+ or −	+ or −	+	+ or −	−	nonspec.	−	−	−
Sinusitis	½	−	−	+ or −	−	local tenderness	−	opaque sinuses	−	−
Optic neuritis	½	−	−	−	−	blindness	−	−	−	−
Glaucoma	½	−	−	−	−	raised intraocular tension	−	−	−	−
ACUTE RECURRENT EPISODES										
Subarachnoid haem. (esp. angioma)	1	+	+	+	+	cer. or cerebellar	occ. focal	−	blood-stained	aneurysm angioma
Cerebral Vascular Insufficiency	½ or 1	−	+ or −	+	−	cer. or b.s.	nonspec.	−	−	vascular stenosis
Intermittent Hydrocephalus	1	−	+ or −	+	+ or −	−	nonspec.	−	−	dilated ventricles

Condition						Signs	EEG	Skull X-ray	L.P.	Radiology
Pressor Reactions of Phaeochromocytoma	1	—	—	—	+	—	nonspec.	—	—	—
Tic Douloureux	½	—	—	—	—	—	—	—	—	—
Cluster	½	+	—	—	—	lacrimation; blocked nostril etc.,	—	—	—	—
Migraine	½ or 1	+	+ or —	+ or —	+ or —	cer. or b.s.	normal or nonspec.	—	—	—
SUBACUTE (days or weeks)										
Subdural Haematoma	½ or 1	—	if coning	+ or —	+ or —	— or c.n. 3 ± paresis	lateralizing	pineal shift	L.P. dangerous	localized
Tumour	½ or 1	—	if coning	+ or —	+ or —	cer. or cerebellar	usually focal	pineal shift	L.P. dangerous	localized
Intracranial Abscess	½ or 1	—	+ or —	+ or —	+	cer. or cerebellar	focal	pineal shift	p.m.n. and lymphocytic usually	localized
Otitic Hydrocephalus	1	—	+ or —	+ or —	+ or —	c.n.6 otitis media	nonspec.	mastoiditis	—	normal or small ventricles
Benign Intracranial Hypertension	1	+ or —	+ or —	+ or —	+ or —	—	nonspec.	—	—	normal or small ventricles
Temporal Arteritis	½ or 1	—	—	—	—	scalp vessels; occ. blindness	—	—	—	—
CHRONIC (months or years)										
Tumour	½ or 1	—	if coning	+ or —	+ or —	cer. or b.s.	normal or focal	pineal shift	L.P. dangerous	localized
Eye Strain	1	—	—	—	—	refractive errors; heterophoria	—	—	—	—
Bite Imbalance	½	—	—	—	—	dental	—	—	—	—
Cervical Spondylosis	½ or 1	—	+ or —	+ or —	+ or —	neck crepitus etc.	—	—	—	—
Psychiatric States	1 > ½	—	—	—	—	—	—	—	—	—
Tension Headache	1 > ½ mild	—	—	—	—	—	—	—	—	—

½ = hemicranial 1 = bilateral headache cer. = cerebral b.s. = brain-stem.

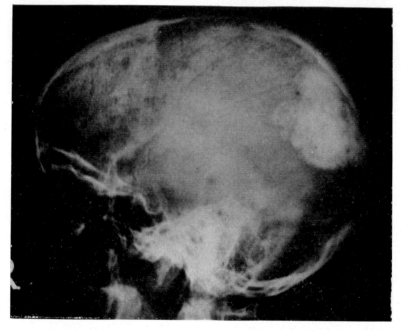

Figure 13.3. An unexpected finding in a routine radiograph of the skull. The patient was an elderly hypertensive woman who had suffered bouts of occipital headache with transient photopsia and hemiparesis, which were thought to be episodes of cerebrovascular insufficiency. Radiography of the skull disclosed a large calcified meningioma, which was removed uneventfully from the occipital region. She is now in her late 70s and remains well some 10 years after the operation

Echoencephalography

The echoencephalograph is a device which is useful in those subjects who are unfortunate enough to have a pineal gland which is uncalcified. The technique is being developed so as to pick up information other than the midline 'echo', such as the position and size of the ventricles and the localization of intracerebral tumours, but at the time of writing other methods give this information more precisely. Echoencephalography is only of value if the recordist is expert in its use.

Brain Scan

Over the past 10 years, brain scanning has matured to become the investigation of choice in screening for brain tumour, and even for cerebral abscess and subdural haematoma if the situation is not urgent (*Figure 13.4*). In addition, the clearance from the ventricular system of radioactive isotope injected into the lumbar CSF is used to confirm the diagnosis of occult hydrocephalus. Dynamic scanning with the gamma camera can also be used to detect inequality of filling of the cerebral hemispheres caused by stenosis or occlusion of the carotid arteries.

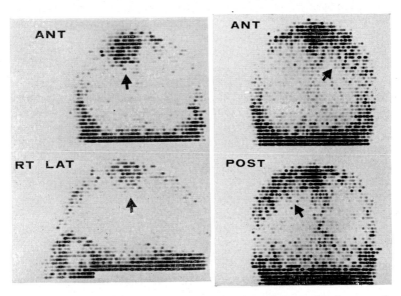

Figure 13.4. (a) Brain-scan showing parasagittal meningioma; (b) the scan of a left subdural haematoma or hygroma

Contrast Radiography

These techniques are probably best limited to neurological units. Carotid and vertebral arteriography, pneumoencephalography, ventriculography and myelography; each has its indications, limitations and hazards, and their judicious use requires some experience.[155b]

CONCLUSIONS

General practitioners have stated to the author their opinion that diagnosis is easy for neurologists because they have so many investigations at their command. His reply is that special investigations are used sparingly in a minority of patients to confirm or deny a specific hypothesis. If a clinical opinion is firmly based it may stand in spite of negative investigations. We all know of patients who were eventually proven to have a cerebral glioma in spite of investigations repeated at intervals of several years with negative results.

Some of the points which contribute to the diagnosis of headache are set out in Table 13.1, which of necessity oversimplifies the clinical problems, but may be of some assistance in clarifying thoughts on a patient presenting with headache. The more time spent in taking the history of a patient with headache, the more likely is the correct diagnosis and solution to emerge, and the more interesting will the patient's problem appear to the doctor.

One patient was referred to the neurological clinic because of curious episodes of blurred vision, vertigo, dysarthria, ataxia, paraesthesiae and occipital headache, for which he had been investigated thoroughly at enormous expense elsewhere. He had accumulated an impressive dossier which he displayed with a mixture of pride and irritation, since no diagnosis had been reached and his attacks continued. The history disclosed one point that had been missed previously—each attack had been preceded by rapid regular palpitations of the heart. Once his paroxysmal tachycardia was controlled by quinidine, his episodes of vertebrobasilar insufficiency disappeared.

Complex investigations are no substitute for the time and thought of the physician.

References

1 Adams, C. W. M., Orton, C. C. and Zilkha, K. J. (1968). 'Arterial catecholamine and enzyme histochemistry in migraine.' *J. Neurol. Neurosurg. Psychiat.* **31,** 50

2 Adams, F. (1841). *The Extant Works of Aretaeus, The Cappadocian,* 294. London; Sydenham Society

3 Adams, F. (1844). *The Seven Books of Paulus Aegineta,* p. 350. London; Sydenham Society

4 Adams, F. (1948). *The Genuine Works of Hippocrates,* pp. 252, 331. London; Sydenham Society

5 Adams, R. D., Fisher, C. M., Hakim, S., Ojemann, R. G. and Sweet, W. H. (1965). 'Symptomatic occult hydrocephalus with "normal" cerebrospinal fluid pressure.' *New Engl. J. Med.* **273,** 117

6 Anderson, B. Jnr., Heyman, A., Whalen, R. E. and Saltzman, H. A. (1965). 'Migraine-like phenomena after decompression from hyperbaric environment.' *Neurology, Minneap.* **15,** 1035

7 Anthony, M., Hinterberger, H. and Lance, J. W. (1967). 'Plasma serotonin in migraine and stress.' *Archs Neurol.* **16,** 544

8 Anthony, M., Hinterberger, H. and Lance, J. W. (1968). 'The possible relationship of serotonin to the migraine syndrome.' *Research and Clinical Studies in Headache* **2,** 29

9 Anthony, M. and Lance, J. W. (1968). 'Indomethacin in migraine.' *Med. J. Aust.* **1,** 56

10 Anthony, M. and Lance, J. W. (1969). 'Monoamine oxidase inhibition in the treatment of migraine.' *Archs Neurol.* **21,** 263

11 Anthony, M. and Lance, J. W. (1971). 'Histamine and serotonin in cluster headache.' *Archs. Neurol.* **25,** 225

12 Anthony, M. and Lance, J. W. (1972). 'A comparative trial of pindolol, clonidine and carbamazepine in the interval therapy of migraine.' *Med. J. Aust.* **1,** 1343

185

[13] Appenzeller, O., Davison, K. and Marshall, J. (1963). 'Reflex vaso-motor abnormalities in the hands of migrainous subjects.' *J. Neurol. Neurosurg. Psychiat.* **26,** 447

[14] Balla, J. I. and Moraitis, S. (1970). 'Knights in armour. A follow-up study of injuries after legal settlement.' *Med. J. Aust.* **2,** 355

[15] Balla, J. I. and Walton, J. N. (1964). 'Periodic migrainous neuralgia.' *Br. med. J.* **1,** 219

[16] Barrie, M. A., Fox, W. R., Weatherall, M. and Wilkinson, M. I. P. (1968). 'Analysis of symptoms of patients with headaches and their response to treatment with ergot derivatives.' *Q. J. Med.* **37,** 319

[17] Barrie, M. and Jowett, A. (1967). 'A pharmacological investigation of cerebro-spinal fluid from patients with migraine.' *Brain* **90,** 785

[18] Basser, L. S. (1969). 'The relation of migraine and epilepsy.' *Brain* **92,** 285

[19] Berde, B. (1971). 'New studies on the circulatory effects of ergot compounds with implications to migraine.' In *Background to Migraine*, p. 66. (Fourth Br. Migraine Symposium.) London; Heinemann

[19a] Bergström, S., Carlson, L. A., and Weeks, J. R. (1968). 'The prostaglandins: a family of biologically active lipids.' *Pharmac. Rev.* **20,** 1

[20] Bianchine, J. R. and Eade, N. R. (1967). 'The effect of 5-hydroxytryptamine on the cotton pellet local inflammatory response in the rat.' *J. Exper. Med.* **125,** 501

[21] Bickerstaff, E. R. (1959). 'The periodic migrainous neuralgia of Wilfred Harris.' *Lancet* **1,** 1069

[22] Bickerstaff, E. R. (1961). 'Impairment of consciousness in migraine.' *Lancet* **2,** 1057

[23] Bille, B. (1962). 'Migraine in school children. *Acta paed., Stockh.* **51,** suppl. 136: 1

[24] Blau, J. N. and Cumings, J. N. (1966). 'Method of precipitating and preventing some migraine attacks.' *Br. med. J.* **2,** 1242

[25] Blau, J. N. and Davis, E. (1970). 'Small blood-vessels in migraine.' *Lancet* **2,** 740

[26] Blend, R. and Bull, J. W. D. (1967). 'The radiological investigation of migraine.' In *Background to Migraine*, p. 1, Ed. by R. Smith. London; Heinemann

[27] Blumenthal, L. S. and Fuchs, M. (1963). 'Current therapy for headache.' *Sth. med. J. Nashville* **56,** 503

[28] Brazil, P. and Friedman, A. P. (1956). 'Craniovascular studies in headache. A report and analysis of pulse volume tracings.' *Neurology, Minneap.* **6,** 96

[29] Brenner, C., Friedman, A. P., Merritt, H. H. and Denny-Brown, D. E. (1944). 'Post-traumatic headache.' *J. Neurosurg.* **6,** 379

[30] Brewis, M., Poskanzer, D. C., Rolland, C. and Miller, H. (1966). 'Neurological disease in an English city.' *Acta. neurol. scand.* **42,** Suppl. 24

31 Broch, A. Hørven, I., Nornes, H., Sjaastad, O. and Tønjum, A. (1970). 'Studies on cerebral and ocular circulation in a patient with cluster headache.' *Headache* **10**, 1

32 Bruyn, G. W. (1968). 'Complicated migraine.' In *Handbook of Clinical Neurology*, Vol. 5, p. 59. Amsterdam; North Holland

33 Bull, J. W. D., Nixon, W. L. B. and Pratt, R. T. C. (1955). 'The radiological criteria and familial occurrence of primary basilar impression.' *Brain* **78**, 229

34 Callaghan, N. (1968). 'The migraine syndrome in pregnancy.' *Neurology, Minneap.* **18**, 197

35 Campbell, D. A., Hay, K. M., and Tonks, E. M. (1951). 'An investigation of the salt and water balance in migraine.' *Br. med. J.* **2**, 1424

36 Carlson, L. A., Ekelund, L-G. and Orö, L. (1968). 'Clinical and metabolic effects of different doses of prostaglandin E in man.' *Acta. med. scand.* **183**, 423

37 Carroll, J. D. (1970). Complicated migraine. In *Kliniske aspekter i Migraeneforskningen*, p. 88. Copenhagen; Nordlundes bogtrykkeri

38 Carroll, P. R. and Glover, W. E. (1972). 'The action of drugs used for the treatment of migraine on the isolated ear artery of the rabbit.' In press

39 Chapman, L. F., Ramos, A. O., Goodell, H., Silverman, G. and Wolff, H. G. (1960). 'A humoral agent implicated in vascular headache of the migrainous type.' *Archs Neurol.* **3**, 223

40 Chawla, J. C. and Falconer, M. A. (1967). 'Glossopharyngeal and vagal neuralgia.' *Br. med. J.* **2**, 529

41 Childs, A. J. and Sweetnam, M. T. (1967). 'A study of 104 cases of migraine.' *Br. J. Ind. Med.* **18**, 234

42 Chorobski, J. and Penfield, W. (1932). 'Cerebral vasodilator nerves and their pathway from the medulla oblongata.' *Archs Neurol. Psychiat., Chicago* **28**, 1257

43 Costen, J. B. (1934). 'A syndrome of ear and sinus symptoms dependent upon disturbed function of the temporomandibular joint.' *Ann. Otol. Rhinol. Lar.* **43**, 1

44 Critchley, M. (1967). 'Migraine from Cappadocia to Queen Square.' In *Background to Migraine*, p. 28, (First Br. Migraine Symposium) London; Heinemann

45 Cumings, J. N. (1971). In *Background to Migraine*, p. 76. (Fourth Br. Migraine Symposium.) London; Heinemann

46 Curran, D. A., Hinterberger, H. and Lance, J. W. (1965). 'Total plasma serotonin, 5-hydroxyindoleacetic acid and p-hydroxy-m-methoxymandelic acid excretion in normal and migrainous subjects.' *Brain* **88**, 997

47 Curran, D. A., Hinterberger, H. and Lance, J. W. (1967). 'Methysergide.' *Research and Clinical Studies in Headache* **1**, 74

48 Curran, D. A. and Lance, J. W. (1964). 'Clinical trial of Methysergide and other preparations in the management of migraine.' *J. Neurol. Neurosurg. Psychiat.* **27,** 463

49 Curzon, G., Barrie, M. and Wilkinson, M. I. P. (1969). 'Relationship between headache and amine changes after administration of reserpine to migrainous patients.' *J. Neurol. Neurosurg. Psychiat.* **32,** 555

50 Curzon, G., Theaker, P. and Phillips, B. (1966). 'Excretion of 5-hydroxyindolyl acetic acid (5HIAA) in migraine.' *J. Neurol. Neurosurg. Psychiat.* **29,** 85

51 Cyriax, J. (1962). 'Text-book of Orthopaedic Medicine.' Vol. 1, p. 193, London; Cassell

52 Dalessio, D. J. (1962). 'On migraine headache: serotonin and serotonin antagonism.' *J. Am. med. Ass.* **181,** 318

53 Dalessio, D. S., Camp, W. A., Goodell, H., Chapman, L. F., Zileli, T., Ramos, A. O., Ehrlich, R., Fortuin, F., Cattell, McK. and Wolff, H. G. (1962). 'Studies on headache. The relevance of the prophylactic action of UML–491 in vascular headache of the migraine type to the pathophysiology of this syndrome.' *Wld. Neurology* **3,** 66

54 Dalessio, D. J., Camp, W. A., Goodell, H. and Wolff, H. G. (1961). 'Studies on headache. The mode of action of UML–491 and its relevance to the nature of vascular headache of the migraine type.' *Archs Neurol.* **4,** 235

55 Dalsgaard-Nielsen, J. (1970). 'Some aspects of the epidemiology of migraine in Denmark.' In *Kliniske Aspekter i migraeneforskningen,* p. 18. Copenhagen; Nordlundes Bogtrykkeri

56 Davis, E. (1967). 'Subarachnoid haemorrhage.' *Med. J. Aust.* **2,** 12

57 De la Lande, I. S., Cannell, V. A. and Waterson, J. G. (1966). 'The interaction of serotonin and noradrenaline on the perfused artery.' *Br. J. Pharmac. Chemother.* **28,** 255

58 Denny-Brown, D. and Yanagisawan (1970). 'The descending trigeminal tract as a mechanism for intersegmental sensory facilitation.' *Trans. Am. Neurol. Ass.* **95,** 129

59 Eckhardt, L. B., McLean, J. M. and Goodell, H. (1943). 'Experimental studies on headache: the genesis of pain from the eye.' *Proc. Ass. Res. nerv. ment. Dis.* **23,** 209

60 Editorial (1964). 'Intracranial hypertension and steroids.' *Lancet* **2,** 1052

61 Ekbom, K. (1970). 'A clinical comparison of cluster headache and migraine.' *Acta neurol. scand.* **46,** suppl. 41: 1

62a Ekbom, K. and Greitz, T. (1970). 'Carotid angiography in cluster headache.' *Acta radiol. (Diagn.)* **10,** 1

62b Ekbom, K. and Lundberg, P. O. (1971). 'Clinical trial of an adrenergic beta-receptor blocking agent in migraine prophylaxis.' *Proc. Scand. Migraine Soc.,* p. 22

63 Elkind, A. H., Friedman, A. P. and Grossman, J. (1964). 'Cutaneous blood flow in vascular headache of the migraine type.' *Neurology, Minneap.* **14,** 24

REFERENCES

[64] Ellard, J. (1970). 'Psychological reactions to compensable injury.' *Med. J. Aust.* **2**, 349

[65] Engel, G. L., Ferris, E. B. and Romano, J. (1945). 'Focal electro-encephalographic changes during the scotomas of migraine.' *Am. J. Med. Sci.* **209**, 650

[66] Every, R. G. (1960). 'The significance of extreme mandibular movements.' *Lancet* **2**, 37

[67] Fang, H. C. H. (1961). 'Cerebral arterial innervations in man.' *Archs Neurol.* **4**, 651

[68] Fay, T. (1937). 'Mechanism of headache.' *Archs Neurol. Psychiat., Chicago* **37**, 471

[69] Fisher, C. M. (1968). 'Headache in cerebrovascular disease.' In *Handbook of Clinical Neurology*, Vol. 5, p. 124. Amsterdam; North Holland

[70] Foley, J. (1955). 'Benign forms of intracranial hypertension— "toxic" and "otitic" hydrocephalus.' *Brain* **78**, 1

[71] Fox, R. H., Goldsmith, R. and Kidd, D. J. (1962). 'Cutaneous vasomotor control in the human head, neck and upper chest.' *J. Physiol. Lond.* **161**, 298

[72] Fox, R. H., Goldsmith, R. Kidd, D. J. and Lewis, G. P. (1961). 'Bradykinin as a vasodilator in man.' *J. Physiol., Lond.* **157**, 589

[73] French, E. B., Lassers, B. W. and Desai, M. G. (1967). 'Reflex vasomotor responses in the hands of migrainous subjects.' *J. Neurol. Neurosurg. Psychiat.* **30**, 276

[74] Friedman, A. P., Finley, K. H., Graham, J. R., Kunkle, E. C., Ostfeld, A. M. and Wolff, H. G. (1962). 'Classification of headache. The Ad Hoc Committee on the Classification of Headache.' *Archs Neurol.* **6**, 173

[75] Friedman, A. P. and Mikropoulos, H. E. (1958). 'Cluster headaches.' *Neurology, Minneap.* **8**, 653

[76] Friedman, A. P., Von Storch, T. J. C. and Merritt, H. H. (1964). 'Migraine and tension headaches. A clinical study of two thousand cases.' *Neurology* **4**, 773

[77] Froese, G. and Burton, A. C. (1957). 'Heat losses from the human head.' *J. appl. Physiol.* **10**, 235

[78] Gardner, J. H., Van den Noort, S. and Horenstein, S. (1967). 'Cerebro vascular disease in young women taking oral contraceptives.' *Neurology, Minneap.* **17**, 297

[79] Goltman, A. M. (1935–6), 'The mechanism of migraine.' *J. Allergy* **7**, 351

[80] Graham, J. R. (1967). 'Cardiac and pulmonary fibrosis during methysergide therapy for headache.' *Am. J. med. Sci.* **254**, 23

[81] Graham, J. R. and Wolff, H. G. (1938). 'Mechanism of migraine headache and action of ergotamine tartrate.' *Archs Neurol. Psychiat., Chicago* **39**, 737

[82] Grant, E. C. G. (1965). 'Relation of arterioles in the endometrium to headache from oral contraceptives.' *Lancet* **1**, 1143

[83] Grimson, B. S., Robinson, S. C., Danford, E. T., Tindall, G. T. and Greenfield, J. C. Jr. (1969). 'Effect of serotonin on internal and external carotid artery flow in the baboon.' *Am. J. Physiol.* **1**, 50

[84] Halmagyi, D. F. and Colebatch, J. H. (1961). 'Serotonin-like cardio-respiratory effects of a serotonin antagonist.' *J. Pharmacol. exp. Ther.* **134**, 47

[85] Hanington, E. (1967). 'Preliminary report on tyramine headache.' *Br. med. J.* **1**, 550

[86] Harris, W. (1936). Ciliary (migrainous) neuralgia and its treatment.' *Br. med. J.* **1**, 457

[87] Hart, C. T. (1967). 'Formed visual hallucinations: A symptom of cranial arteritis.' *Br. med. J.* **2**, 643

[88] Hauptmann, A. (1946). 'Capillaries in the finger nail fold in patients with neurosis, epilepsy and migraine.' *Archs Neurol. Psychiat., Chicago* **56**, 631

[89] Hertzman, A. B. and Roth, L. W. (1942). 'The absence of vaso-constrictor reflexes in the forehead circulation. Effects of cold.' *Am. J. Physiol.* **136**, 692

[90] Heyck, H. (1969). 'Pathogenesis of migraine.' In Research and Clinical Studies in Headache. Vol. 2., p. 1. Basel and New York; Karger

[91] Hilton, J. (1950). *Rest and Pain*, p. 77. Ed. by E. W. Walls, and E. E. Philipp. London; Bell

[92] Hockaday, J. M., Macmillan, A. L. and Whitty, C. W. M. (1967). 'Vasomotor-reflex response in idiopathic and hormone-dependent migraine.' *Lancet* **1**, 1023

[93] Hockaday, J. M., Williamson, D. H. and Whitty, C. W. M. (1971). 'Blood glucose levels and fatty acid metabolism in migraine related to fasting.' *Lancet* **1**, 1153

[94a] Horton, B. J., MacLean, A. R. and Craig, W. McK. (1939). 'A new syndrome of vascular headache: results of treatment with histamine: preliminary report.' *Proc. Staff Meet. Mayo Clin.* **14**, 257

[94b] Horton, E. W. (1969). 'Hypothesis on physiological roles of prosta-glandins.' *Physiol. Rev.* **49**, 122

[95] Hudgson, P., Foster, J. B. and Newell, D. J. (1967). 'Controlled trial of Demigran in the prophylaxis of migraine.' *Br. med. J.* **1**, 91

[96] Hunter, C. R. and Mayfield, F. H. (1949). 'Role of the upper cervical roots in the production of pain in the head.' *Am. J. Surg.* **78**, 743

[97] Jacobsen, E. (1938). *Progressive relaxation.* Illinois; Univ. Chicago Press

[98] Jefferson, A. (1956). 'A Clinical correlation between encephalopathy and papilloedema in Addison's disease.' *J. Neurol. Neurosurg. Psychiat.* **19**, 21

[99] Johnson, R. T., Johnson, K. P. and Edmonds, C. J. (1967). 'Virus-induced hydrocephalus: development of aqueductal stenosis in hamsters after mumps infection.' *Science* **157**, 1066

[100] Keele, C. A. (1964). *Substances Producing Pain and Itch.* London; Arnold

[101] Kerr, F. W. L. (1961a). 'Trigeminal and cervical volleys.' *Archs Neurol.* **5,** 171

[102] Kerr, F. W. L. (1961b). 'A mechanism to account for frontal headache in cases of posterior fossa tumours.' *J. Neurosurg.* **18,** 605

[103] Kerr, F. W. L. (1967). 'Evidence for a peripheral etiology of trigeminal neuralgia.' *J. Neurosurg.* **26,** 168

[104] Kimball, R. W., Friedman, A. P. and Vallejo, E. (1960). 'Effect of serotonin in migraine patients.' *Neurology, Minneap.* **10,** 107

[105] Kimball, R. W. and Goodman, M. A. (1966). 'Effects of reserpine on amino-acid excretion in patients with migraine.' *J. Neurol. Neurosurg. Psychiat.* **29,** 190

[106] Klee, A. (1968). *A Clinical Study of Migraine with Particular Reference to the Most Severe Cases.* Copenhagen; Munksgaard

[107] Kunkle, E. C. (1959). 'Acetylcholine in the mechanism of headaches of the migraine type.' *Arch. Neurol. Psychiat., Chicago* **84,** 135

[108] Kunkle, E. C. (1963). 'Headache mechanisms, with particular reference to migraine.' *Neurology Minneap.* **13,** 1

[109] Kunkle, E. C. and Anderson, W. B. (1961). 'Significance of minor eye signs in headache of migraine type.' *Archs Ophthal. Chicago* **65,** 504

[110] Kunkle, E. C., Pfeiffer, J. B., Wilhoit, W. M. and Lamrick, L. W. (1954). 'Recurrent brief headaches in "cluster" pattern.' *N. Carol. med. J.* **15,** 510

[111] Kuntz, A. (1934). 'Nerve fibers of spinal and vagus origin associated with the cephalic sympathetic nerves.' *Ann. Otol. Rhinol. Lar.* **43,** 50

[112] Kuntz, A., Hoffman, H. H. and Napolitano, L. M. (1957). 'Cephalic sympathetic nerves.' *Archs surg.* **75,** 108

[113] Lance, J. W. and Anthony, M. (1966). 'Some clinical aspects of migraine.' *Archs Neurol.* **15,** 356

[114] Lance, J. W. and Anthony, M. (1968). 'Clinical trial of a new serotonin antagonist, BC105, in migraine.' *Med. J. Aust.* **1,** 54

[115] Lance, J. W. and Anthony, M. (1971). 'Thermographic studies in vascular headache.' *Med. J. Aust.* **1,** 240

[116] Lance, J. W. and Anthony, M. (1971). 'Migrainous neuralgia or cluster headache?' *J. Neurol. Sci.* **13,** 401

[117] Lance, J. W. and Anthony, M. (1972). 'The cephalgias.' In *The Cellular and Molecular Basis of Neurologic Disease.* Ed. by S. H. Appel and E. S. Goldensohn. Philadelphia; Lea and Febiger

[118] Lance, J. W., Anthony, M. and Gonski, A. (1967). 'Serotonin, the carotid body and cranial vessels in migraine.' *Archs Neurol.* **16,** 553

[119] Lance, J. W., Anthony, M. and Somerville, B. (1970). 'Comparative trial of serotonin antagonists in the management of migraine.' *Br. med. J.* **2,** 327

[120] Lance, J. W. and Curran, D. A. (1964). 'Treatment of Chronic tension headache.' *Lancet* **1**, 1236

[121] Lance, J. W., Curran, D. A. and Anthony, M. (1965). 'Investigations into the mechanism and treatment of chronic headache.' *Med. J. Aust.* **2**, 909

[122] Lance, J. W., Fine, R. D. and Curran, D. A. (1963). 'An evaluation of methysergide in the prevention of migraine and other vascular headaches.' *Med. J. Aust.* **1**, 814

[123] Lashley, K. S. (1941). 'Patterns of cerebral integration indicated by the scotomas of migraine.' *Archs Neurol. Psychiat., Chicago* **46**, 331

[124] Lennox, W. G. and Lennox, M. A. (1960). *Epilepsy and Related Disorders*, Vol. 1, p. 438. London; Churchill

[125] Leviton, A. and Camenga, D. (1969). 'Migraine associated with hyper-pre-beta lipoproteinemia.' *Neurology* **19**, 963

[126] Lim, R. K. S., Miller, D. G., Guzman, F., Rodgers, D. W., Rogers, R. W., Wang, S. K., Chao, P. Y. and Shih, T. Y. (1967). 'Pain and analgesia evaluated by the intraperitoneal bradykinin-evoked pain method in man.' *Clin. Pharmac. Ther.* **8**, 521

[127] Lund, F. (1957). 'Studies on the shape of the temporal artery pulsations in vascular headache, particularly migraine.' *Acta med. scand.* **158**, 21

[128] Lundberg, P. O. (1962). 'Migraine prophylaxis with progestogens.' *Acta endocr., Copenh.* **40**, suppl. 68, 5

[129] Macmillan, A. L. and Hockaday, J. (1966). 'The effect of migraine and ergot upon reflex vasodilatation to radiant heating.' Proc. 4th Europ. Conf. on Micro-circulation, p. 343. Basel and New York; Karger

[130] Marshall, W. H. (1959). 'Spreading cortical depression of Leão.' *Physiol. Rev.* **39**, 239

[131] Martin, M. J. and Rome, H. P. (1967). 'Muscle-contraction headache: therapeutic aspects.' In *Research and Clinical Studies in Headache* **1**, 205

[132] Martin, M. J., Rome, H. P. and Swenson, W. M. (1967). 'Muscle-contraction headache: a psychiatric review.' *Research and Clinical Studies in Headache* **1**, 184

[133] McAlpine, D., Lumsden, C. E. and Acheson, E. D. (1965). *Multiple Sclerosis. A Reappraisal.* Edinburgh and London; Livingstone

[134] McNaughton, F. L. (1937). 'The innervation of the intracranial blood vessels and dural sinuses.' *Proc. Ass. Res. nerv. ment. Dis.* **18**, 178

[135] Meyer, J. S., Yoshida, K. and Sakamoto, K. (1967). 'Autonomic control of cerebral blood flow measured by electromagnetic flowmeters.' *Neurology, Minneap.* **17**, 638

[136] Miller, H. (1961). 'Accident neurosis.' *Br. med. J.* **1**, 919, 992

[137] Milner, P. M. (1958). 'Note on a possible correspondence between the scotomas of migraine and spreading depression of Leão.' *EEG clin. Neurophysiol.* **10**, 705

[138] Nieman, E. A. and Hurwitz, L. J. (1961). 'Ocular sympathetic palsy in periodic migrainous neuralgia.' *J. Neurol. Neurosurg. Psychiat.* **24**, 369

[139] O'Brien, M. D. (1970). 'Cerebral cortex perfusion rates measured in carotid artery distribution in the migraine syndrome.' In *Kliniske Aspekter i Migraeneforskningen*, p. 40. Copenhagen; Nordlundes Bogtrykkeri

[140] Oka, M. (1950). 'Experimental study on the vasodilator innervation of the face.' *Med. J. Osaka Univ.* **2**, 109

[141] Olivecrona, H. (1947). 'Notes on the surgical treatment of migraine.' *Acta. med. scand. Suppl.* 196, 229

[142] Onel, Y., Friedman, A. P. and Grossman, J. (1961). 'Muscle blood flow studies in muscle-contraction headaches.' *Neurology, Minneap.* **11**, 935

[143] Ostfeld, A. M. (1960). 'Migraine headache. Its physiology and biochemistry.' *J. Am. med. Ass.* **174**, 110

[144] Ostfeld, A. M., Chapman, L. F., Goodell, H. and Wolff, H. G. (1957). 'Summary of evidence concerning a noxious agent active locally during migraine headache.' *Psychosom. Med.* **19**, 199

[145] Ostfeld, A. M., Reis, D. J. and Wolff, H. G. (1957). 'Studies on headache: bulbar conjunctival ischemia and muscle-contraction headache.' *Archs Neurol. Psychiat., Chicago* **77**, 113

[146] Ostfeld, A. M. and Wolff, H. G. (1955). 'Studies on headache: arterenol (norepinephrine) and vascular headache of the migraine type.' *Archs Neurol. Psychiat., Chicago* **74**, 131

[147] Paulley, J. W. and Hughes, J. P. (1960). 'Giant-cell arteritis, or arteritis of the aged.' *Br. med. J.* **2**, 1562

[148] Pearce, J. (1969). *Migraine, Clinical Features, Mechanisms and Management.* Springfield; Thomas

[149] Penfield, W. (1932). 'Operative treatment of migraine and observations on the mechanism of vascular pain.' *Trans. Am. Acad. Ophthal. Oto-lar.* **37**, 50

[150] Pickering, G. W. and Hess, W. (1933–4). 'Observations on the mechanism of headache produced by histamine.' *Clin. Sci.* **1**, 77

[151] Pluvinage, R. (1970). 'Headache, including migraine, and oral contraception.' In *Background to Migraine*, p. 150. (Third Br. Migraine Symposium.) London; Heinemann

[152] Rawson, M. D., Liversedge, L. A. and Goldfarb, G. (1966). 'Treatment of acute retrobulbar neuritis with corticotrophin.' *Lancet* **2**, 1044

[153] Ray, B. S. and Wolff, H. G. (1940). 'Experimental studies on headache. Pain sensitive structures of the head and their significance in headache.' *Archs Surg.* **41**, 813

[154] Redisch, W. and Pelzer, R. H. (1943). 'Capillary studies in migraine: effect of ergotamine tartrate and water diuresis.' *Am. Heart. J.* **26**, 598

[155a] Riley, H. A. (1932). 'Migraine.' *Bull. Neur. Inst. N.Y.* **2**, 429

193

o

[155b] Robertson, E. G. (1972). 'The investigation of headache.' In *Research and Clinical Studies in Headache*, 3. Basel and New York; Karger

[156] Robinson, B. W. (1958). 'Histaminic cephalgia.' *Medicine, Baltimore* **37**, 161

[157] Romberg, M. H. (1840). *A Manual of Nervous Diseases of Man.* Trans. by E. H. Sieveking. London; Sydenham Society

[158] Rompel, H. and Bauermeister, P. W. (1970). 'Aetiology of migraine and prevention with carbamazepine (Tegretol): results of a double-blind crossover study.' *S. Afr. med. J.* **44**, 75

[159] Rowbotham, G. F. (1949). 'The surgical treatment of migraine.' *IVe Congrès Neurologique International.* Paris; Masson. **1**, 147

[160] Rooke, E. D. (1968). 'Benign exertional headache.' *Med. Clins. N. Am.* **52**, 801

[161] Russell, D. S. (1949). 'Observations on the pathology of Hydrocephalus.' *M.R.C. Special Report No. 265*, London

[162a] Sandler, M. (1972). 'Migraine: a pulmonary disease?' *Lancet* **1**, 618.

[162b] Sandler, M., Youdim, M. B. H., Southgate, J. and Hanington, E. (1970). 'The role of tyramine in migraine: Some possible biochemical mechanisms.' In *Background to Migraine*, p. 103. (Third Br. Migraine Symposium.) London; Heinemann

[163] Schottstaedt, W. W. and Wolff, H. G. (1955). 'Variations in fluid and electrolyte excretion in association with vascular headache of the migraine type.' *Archs Neurol. Psychiat., Chicago* **73**, 158

[164] Schumacher, G. A. and Wolff, H. G. (1941). 'Experimental studies on headache: contrast of histamine headache with headache of migraine and that associated with hypertension.' *Archs Neurol. Psychiat., Chicago* **45**, 199

[165] Schwartz, F. D. and Dunea, G. (1966). 'Progression of retroperitoneal fibrosis despite cessation of treatment with methysergide.' *Lancet* **1**, 955

[166] Selby, G. and Lance, J. W. (1960). 'Observations on 500 cases of migraine and allied vascular headache.' *J. Neurol. Neurosurg. Psychiat.* **23**, 23

[167] Sicuteri, F. (1962). 'L'acido vanilmandelico (VMA) il maggior metabolita urinario della catecolamine.' *Sett. med.* **50**, 227

[168] Sicuteri, F. (1963). 'Mast cells and their active substances. Their role in the pathogenesis of migraine.' *Headache* **3**, 86

[169] Sicuteri, F. (1967). 'Vasoneuroactive substances and their implication in vascular pain.' *Research and Clinical Studies in Headache* **1**, 6

[170] Sicuteri, F., Fanciullacci, M. and Anselmi, B. (1963). 'Bradykinin release and inactivation in man.' *Int. Archs Allergy. appl. Immun.* **22**, 77

[171] Sicuteri, F., Franchi, G. and Del Bianco, P. L. (1967). 'An antaminic drug, BC105, in the prophylaxis of migraine.' *Int. Archs Allergy. appl. Immun.* **31**, 78

172 Sicuteri, F., Michelacci, S. and Anselmi, B. (1964). 'Individuazione della proprietà vasoattive ed antiemicraniche dell' indomethacin, nuovo antiflogistico di derivazione indolica.' *Sett. med.* **52,** 335

173 Sicuteri, F., Ricci, M., Monfardini, R. and Ficini, M. (1957). 'Experimental headache with endogenous histamine.' *Acta allerg.* **11,** 188

174 Sicuteri, F., Testi, A. and Anselmi, B. (1961). 'Biochemical investigations in headache: increase in hydroxyindoleacetic acid excretion during migraine attacks.' *Int. Archs Allergy. appl. Immun.* **19,** 55

175 Sjaastad, O. (1970). 'Kinin- and histamine-investigations in vascular headache.' In *Kliniske Aspekter i Migraeneforskningen,* p. 61. Copenhagen; Nordlundes Bogtrykkeri

176a Sjaastad, O. and Stensrud, P. (1969). 'Appraisal of BC105 in migraine prophylaxis.' *Acta. neurol. scand.* **45,** 594

176c Sjaastad, O. and Stensrud, P. (1971). 2-(2,6-dichlorophenylamino)-2-imidazoline hydrochloride (ST155 or Catapressan) as a prophylactic agent against migraine. *Acta neurol. scand.* **47,** 120

176b Sjaastad, O. and Stensrud, P. (1971). Clinical trial of a beta-blocking agent in migraine prophylaxis. *Proc. Scand. Migraine Soc.,* p. 27

177 Skinhøj, E. (1970). 'Determination of regional cerebral blood flow within the internal carotid system during the migraine attack.' In *Kliniske Aspekter i Migraeneforskningen,* p. 43. Copenhagen; Nordlundes Bogtrykkeri

178 Sluder, G. (1910). 'The syndrome of sphenopalatine-ganglion neurosis.' *Am. J. med. Sci.* **140,** 868

179 Somerville, B. W. (1971). 'Daily variations in plasma levels of estradiol and progesterone during the normal menstrual cycle.' *Am. J. Obstet. Gynec.* **111,** 419

180 Somerville, B. W. (1971). 'The role of progesterone in menstrual migraine.' *Neurology, Minneap.* **21,** 853

181 Somerville, B. W. (1972). 'The role of estradiol withdrawal in the etiology of menstrual migraine.' *Neurology, Minneap.* **22.** In press

182 Somerville, B. W. (1972). 'A study of migraine in pregnancy.' *Neurology, Minneap.* **22.** In press

183 Southren, A. L. and Christoff, N. (1962). 'Cerebrospinal fluid serotonin in brain tumour and other neurological disorders determined by a spectrophotofluorometric technique.' *J. Lab. clin. Med.* **59,** 320

184 Stanford, E. and Greene, R. (1970). 'A case of migraine cured by treatment of Conn's syndrome.' In *Background to Migraine,* p. 53. (Third Br. Migraine Symposium.) London; Heinemann

185 Susman, E. (1929). 'Migraine ophthalmoplegique (Charcot).' *Med. J. Aust.* **11,** 793

186 Sutherland, J. M. and Eadie, M. J. (1972). 'Cluster headache.' In *Research and Clinical Studies in Headache,* **3.** Basel and New York; Karger. In press

[187] Sutherland, J. M., Tyrer, J. H., Eadie, M. J., Leaming, D. B., Courtice, B. and Leggett, C. A. C. (1966). 'Neurological presentations of insulin secreting tumours of the pancreas.' *Aust. Ann. Med.* **15,** 136

[188] Sweetnam, M. T. (1961). 'An enquiry into the treatment of migraine.' *J. Coll. gen. Practnrs. Res. Newsl.* **4,** 538

[189] Symonds, C. P. (1956). 'A particular variety of headache.' *Brain* **79,** 217

[190] Symonds, C. P. (1956). 'Cough headache.' *Brain* **79,** 557

[191] Tandon, R. N., Sur, B. K. and Nath, K. (1969). 'Effect of reserpine injections in migrainous and normal control subjects, with estimations of urinary 5-hydroxyindoleacetic acid.' *Neurology* **19,** 1073

[192] Taylor, A. R. (1967). 'Post-concussional sequelae.' *Br. med. J.* **2,** 67

[193] Thonnard-Neumann, E. (1969). 'Some interrelationships of vaso active substances and basophilic leukocytes in migraine headache.' *Headache* **9,** 130

[194] Thonnard-Neumann, E. and Taylor, W. L. (1968). 'The basophilic leukocyte and migraine.' *Headache* **8,** 98

[195] Tunis, M. M. and Wolff, H. G. (1952). 'Analysis of cranial artery pulse waves in patients with vascular headache of the migraine type.' *Am. J. med. Sci.* **224,** 565

[196] Tunis, M. M. and Wolff, H. G. (1953). 'Studies on headache: long-term observations of the reactivity of the cranial arteries in subjects with vascular headache of the migraine type.' *Archs Neurol. Psychiat., Chicago* **70,** 551

[197] Tunis, M. M. and Wolff, H. G. (1954). 'Studies on headache. Cranial artery vasoconstriction and muscle-contraction headache.' *Archs Neurol. Psychiat., Chicago* **71,** 425

[198] Vail, H. H. (1932). 'Vidian neuralgia.' *Ann. Otol. Rhinol. Lary.* **41,** 837

[199] Von Reis, G., Lund, F. and Sahlgren, E. (1957). 'Experimental histamine headache.' *Acta med. scand.* **157,** 451

[200] Walker, C. H. (1959). 'Migraine and its relationship to hypertension.' *Br. med. J.* **2,** 1430

[201] Wall, P. D. and Pribram, K. H. (1950). 'Trigeminal neurotomy and blood pressure responses from stimulation of lateral cerebral cortex of *Macaca mulata.' J. Neurophysiol.* **13,** 409

[202] Walton, J. N. (1956). *Subarachnoid Haemorrhage.* Edinburgh and London; Livingstone

[203] Waters, W. E. (1970). 'Controlled clinical trial of ergotamine tartrate.' *Br. med. J.* **1,** 325

[204] Waters, W. E. and O'Connor, P. J. (1970). 'The clinical validation of a headache questionnaire.' In *Background to Migraine*, p. 1. (Third Br. Migraine Symposium.) London; Heinemann

[205] Webb, H. E. and Lascelles, R. G. (1962). 'Treatment of facial and head pain associated with depression.' *Lancet* **1,** 355

[206] Weber, R. B. and Reinmuth, O. M. (1971). 'The treatment of migraine with propranalol.' *Neurology* **21**, 404

[207] Wennerholm, M. (1961). 'Postural vascular reactions in cases of migraine and related vascular headaches.' *Acta med. scand.* **169,** 131

[208] White, J. C. and Smithwick, R. H. (1944). *The Autonomic Nervous System*, p. 255. London; Kimpton

[209] White, J. and Sweet, W. (1955). *Pain. Its Mechanism and Neurosurgical Control.* Springfield; Thomas

[210] Whitty, C. W. M. (1953). 'Familial hemiplegic migraine.' *J. Neurol. Neurosurg. Psychiat.* **16,** 172

[211] Whitty, C. W. M. and Hockaday, J. M. (1968). 'Migraine. A follow-up study of 92 patients.' *Br. med. J.* **1,** 735

[212] Whitty, C. W. M., Hockaday, J. M. and Whitty, M. M. (1966). 'The effect of oral contraceptives on migraine.' *Lancet* **1,** 856

[213] Wilkinson, M. (1970). 'The use of clonidine in migraine.' International Migraine Headache Symposium, Florence

[214] Wolff, H. G. (1963). *Headache and Other Head Pain.* London and New York, Oxford Univ. Press

[215] Woodforde, J. M., Dwyer, B., McEwan, B. W., De Wilde, F. W., Bleasel, K., Connelly, T. J. and Ho, C. Y. (1965). 'Treatment of post-herpetic neuralgia.' *Med. J. Aust.* **2,** 869

[216] Wurzel, M., Blair, D. C., Zweifach, B. W., Craig, L. C. and Taylor, W. I. (1967). 'Blood-borne factors affecting vascular tone.' *Experientia* **23,** 486

[217] Zaimis, E. and Hanington, E. (1969). 'A possible pharmacological approach to migraine.' *Lancet* **2,** 298

INDEX

Abscess
  cerebral, 65, 66
  intracranial, 65,
Accident neurosis, 71
Acetylcholine, migraine, in, 120
ACTH, 63
Addison's disease, 52, 174
Adenosine triphosphate, 125, 130
Adrenaline-noradrenaline balance,
  phaeochromocytoma, in, 53
β-Adrenergic blocking agents,
  migraine, in, 141, 150
Albuminuria, 35
Alcohol precipitating headache,
  24, 111, 161
Aldosteronism and migraine, 111
Allergy, relationship to migraine, 97
Amitriptyline, 70, 88, 89
Aneurysm, relationship to migraine,
  37, 38
Angiography, carotid, 2, 41
Angioma, 38
Anticonvulsants, migraine, in, 142
Antidepressant drugs, 88
A.P.C. powders, 25
Aretaeus on migraine, 11
'Armchair sign' in examination for
  tension headache, 77
Arteries
  cerebral, pain from, 2
  extracranial, pain from, 4
  temporal, pulsation in migraine,
  112
  vertebral, nerve plexus, 4
Arteritis, temporal, 57

Aspirin, 25, 80, 84

Barometric pressure changes, 24, 117
Beta adrenergic blocking agents,
  migraine, in, 141, 150
Blood
  count, in investigation of
  headache, 58, 175
  pressure, arterial, increased, 111,
  112
  venous, increased, 49
  vessels, changes in migraine, 101
  extracranial, inflammation, 56
Bradykinin
  migraine, and, 120
  antagonists, treatment of
  migraine, in, 143
  pain, and, 84
Brain
  abscess headache, 1, 7, 65
  oedema, 1, 50
  scan, investigation of headache,
  in, 182
  tumour headache, 1, 7, 23, 41–46,
  173, 174

Caffeine habituation headache, 52
Carbamazepine
  control of migraine, in, 142, 168
  tic douloureux, in, 60
Caries, dental, pain from, 67
Carotid body
  removal, treatment of migraine,
  in, 119
Carotid nerve plexus, 2

199